KETO AFTER 50

RESTART YOUR METABOLISM AND BOOST YOUR ENERGY; THE ULTIMATE 2020 GUIDE TO KETOGENIC DIET FOR SENIORS OVER 50 | LOSE WEIGHT & CUT CHOLESTEROL IN A HEALTHY WAY |

MICHELLE CLARITY

Copyright © 2020 by Michelle Clarity

All rights reserved. No part of this book may be reproduced or used in any manner without written permission of the copyright owner except for the use of quotations in a book review.

First paperback edition March 2020

Book design by Michelle Claritu

For More Info:

michelle.clarity@gmail.com

Table of Contents

Introduction 9
   History of the Ketogenic Diet 9

Chapter 1: What is Ketogenic? 13
   The Science Behind It 13
   What is Ketosis? 15
   Why Is It Important for People Over 50? 16
   Body Changes after 50 19
      Your Metabolic Rate Slows Down 19
      Your Muscle Power Decreases 20
      Your Bones Become More Brittle 20
      Your Excess Weight Increases 20
   Benefits of the Keto Diet for People over 50 21

Chapter 2: Keto for Women Over 50 24
   Keto: The Need of the Hour 26
      Menopause 27
      Heart Diseases 29
      Diabetes Control 29
      And so Much More! 29
      All Set to Begin? 30

Chapter 3: Keto for Men Over 50 31
   50 Marks the Start of Troubles 32
      Helping You Live Longer 34
      Good Under the Sheets 35
      Strengthening the Bones 36
      Keto Helps to Prevent Certain Cancers 37
      Some Side Effects You Should Know 37

The side effects include:..38

Chapter 4: Keto for Women vs. Men...40

Why Keto for 50+? 43

Chapter 5: What Is the Keto Flu?..47

Signs & Symptoms of the Keto Flu 47

Causes of the Keto Flu..48

    Keto Adaption..49

    Carbohydrate Withdrawal...49

    Lack of Micronutrients 50

    Electrolyte Imbalance..51

How to Get Over the Keto Flu 52

    Drink Up and Stay Hydrated 52

    Think Electrolytes..53

    Increase Fats..54

    Work it Out 56

Preventing the Keto Flu..56

    Follow the Diet 56

    The Power of Sleep 57

    Supplement...57

Chapter 6: Health Benefits of the Ketogenic Diet 58

Brain Benefits 58

Heart Disease 59

Fight Cancer 60

Improve Sleep and Energy Levels..60

Decrease Inflammation...61

Gastrointestinal and Gallbladder Health..62

Improved Kidney Function 62

Improved Women's Health..63

Improved Endurance and Muscle Gain 64
Weight Loss 65
Increased Metabolic Health 65

Chapter 7: Keto Side Effects and How to Solve Them 67
Long Term Side Effects 67
Keto Flu 68
    Constipation or Diarrhea 72

Chapter 8: Most Common Keto Diet Mistakes You Should Know .. 73
The 9 Common Mistakes Beginners Do During Keto 73
Give up before you stop ketosis 73
    Lack of salt and minerals 74
    Consume too much protein 74
    Insufficient fat consumption 75
    Consume bad quality food 75
    Do not introduce the right amount of fiber 75
    Eat raw vegetables 75
    Consume the highest protein load at dinner 76
    Not drinking enough 76
Ketogenic Foods 77
Best Foods to Fit into the Keto Diet for Older Adults 77
    Seafood 77
    Vegetables 78
    Cheese 78
    Avocados 78
    Meat and Poultry 78
    Eggs 79
    Coconut Oil 79
    Plain Greek Yogurt and Cottage Cheese 79

- Olive Oil...79
- Nuts and Seeds..80
- Berries..80
- Butter and Cream..80
- Shirataki Noodles..80
- Unsweetened Coffee and Tea...80
- Dark Chocolate and Cocoa Powder 81
- Allowed Product List..81
  - Meat and Poultry..81
  - Seafood..81
  - Vegetables 82
  - Dairy Products 83
  - Berries..84
  - Nuts and Seeds..84
  - Coconut and Olive Oils...85
  - Low-Carb Drinks..85
- Prohibited Product List..86
- Keto diet Menu for The Beginner: Understanding SKD, TKD and CKD..87
  - Standard-SKD 88
  - Targeted-TKD...88
  - Cyclical-CKD..88

Chapter 9: Fitness and Exercise: How to Lose Weight and Alleviate the Symptoms of Menopause 89

- Physical activity strengthens muscles and bones..............................92
- Physical activity in the gym: recommendations................................92
- Physical activity to prevent or treat various problems 93
- Ketogenic Diet FAQs 95
  - Why are you here? 95

Is there such a thing as too much fat? 95

How much weight can you lose? 96

Should I be counting calories? 96

Primary Keto Guidelines—the Do's and Don'ts of 98

Do Consult Your Doctor Beforehand 99

Do Eat Less Than 50 Grams of Carbohydrates 99

Do Increase Your Fat Intake 100

Do Eat the Good Kind of Meat..100

Do Avoid Excessive Exercise 100

The End Goal: Achieving Ketosis 101

Chapter 10: Keto Recipes 102

Banana Waffles...102

Keto Cinnamon Coffee..104

Keto Waffles and Blueberries 105

Baked Avocado Eggs 106

Mushroom Omelet 108

Chocolate Sea Salt Smoothie 110

Zucchini Lasagna 111

Vegan Keto Scramble...113

Keto Snacks Recipes...115

Parmesan Cheese Strips 115

Peanut Butter Power Granola..116

Homemade Graham Crackers 118

Keto No-Bake Cookies 120

Swiss Cheese Crunchy Nachos 121

Keto Dessert Recipes 123

Keto Cheesecake with Blueberries 123

Keto Lemon Ice Cream 125

Peanut Butter Balls 127

Keto Cake Donuts 128

Chocolate Coconut Candies 130

Chicken Wings Black Pepper with Sesame Seeds 132

Spicy Chicken Curry Samosa 134

Garlic Chicken Balls 136

Savory Chicken Fennel 138

Spicy Glazed Pork Loaf 140

Spicy Keto Chicken Wings 142

Cilantro and Lime Creamed Chicken 144

Cheesy Ham Quiche 146

Loaded Cauliflower Rice 148

Super Herbed Fish 150

Beef Rib Steak with Parsley Lemon Butter 152

Marinated Flank Steak with Beef Gravy 154

Buttery Beef Loin and Cheese Sauce 156

Chapter 11: Meal Plan 158

Ketogenic Diet Meal Plan 159

Weekly Meal Plan (4 Week Meal Plan) 159

Conclusion 162

Introduction

Before starting any diet, it is crucial that you understand the history behind it. As you well know, there are many diets on the market in the modern age. The right question you need to ask for yourself is, is the Ketogenic Diet right for you? Luckily for all of us, the Ketogenic Diet can help a wide range of individuals, whether you are young, older, or somewhere in between!

History of the Ketogenic Diet

The Ketogenic Diet first began in the 1920s and 30s. Initially, it was a popular therapy for individuals who had epilepsy. At the very beginning, the Ketogenic Diet was first developed to provide an alternative to fasting, which also worked well for epilepsy therapy.

While the diet did work for a while for these patients, it was eventually abandoned when modern medicine came around and was able to help a majority of patients with their symptoms. However, there were still approximately 30% of patients where the medication did not work, and the diet was re-introduced to help these individuals.

In 1921, it was an endocrinologist known as Rollin Woodyatt that was one of the first to notice the three water-soluble compounds that are produced in the liver when we are starved from carbohydrates. These three compounds are what we now know as ketone bodies. It was at this point, an individual from the Mayo Clinic known as Russel Wilder would call this "starvation from carbohydrates" as the Ketogenic Diet!

It is imperative to note that the ketogenic diet for people in their 30s is different from those in their 50s. The main difference is in the amount of energy required to do various activities. In your younger years, you will need more energy to allow you to carry out your activities easily. There is solid evidence that a ketogenic diet can reduced seizures. Since it has neuroprotective features, your brain cells will be replenished, and you will not experience memory loss quickly. Some studies suggest that a ketogenic diet can help in preventing disorders such as Alzheimer's, sleep disorders, autism, and Parkinson's disease. Weight loss is the most important aspect of a ketogenic diet, and you can easily lose weight with the ketogenic diet. It will help in improving blood sugar levels as well as rejuvenating your brain cells as well as give you a feel-good mood.

Although the diet is solely based on fats and proteins, you should try and take fats and proteins that are healthy. Avoid processed salty foods as well as fats with low-density lipoproteins. Eating healthy is the first way of building a better immune system and a better mood throughout the day. Choose the ketogenic diet and enjoy the benefits that come with it.

A ketogenic diet provides your body with premium fuel, which is fat, and it makes you feel fitter, stronger, and younger. You can achieve all this by following a diet that will burn away excess fat and take your body and health to a whole new level. So why is the ketogenic diet the most preferred type of diet for people after 50?

Ketogenic diet is considered as a miracle diet because it will turn around your health and allow your cells to rejuvenate quickly. The body has different metabolic pathways that are essential in the production of energy. However, some are used more than others because of cellular preference. The main source of energy in the body is usually glucose, and this is the simplest form of sugar.

Most of the sugar that we consume is a pure form of glucose; on the other hand, some of the carbohydrates can be broken down into glucose. When the body runs low on glucose, it can break down fats into energy, and this is a process called gluconeogenesis. Besides, the body can run on other energy sources such as free fatty acids and ketones. However, it is important to note that the body will only run on alternative sources of energy once glucose is depleted in the system. The depletion of glucose in the body usually results from fasting or eating a diet that is low in carbohydrates.

The glucose depletion process can take anywhere from 24 to 36 hours, although this process can be sped up by carrying out various forms of exercises. As the glucose reserves get depleted, the body will compensate for the energy needs by burning free fatty acids.

As the diet continues to grow in popularity, there is more research being performed on the Ketogenic Diet by the day! With science-backed evidence, you can follow the diet and know for a fact that it is going to work.

Welcome to your first Ketogenic Diet Science lesson! One of the best parts of the Ketogenic Diet is the fact that it is based around a natural process that your body already has! The key to success is fueling your body correctly instead of stuffing it with overly-processed junk. In this guide, you will learn everything you need to know from what to eat when to eat and how to get into the best shape of your life.

Chapter 1: What is Ketogenic?

Keto, short for ketogenic, is a form of diet that primarily focuses on cutting down carbs and increasing the protein intake of a person. The idea is that you cut back and remove all the easy-to-digest carbs from your regular intake such as sugar, white bread, sodas, and so on. In return, you are left with a healthy dose of good fats, a sufficient amount of protein, and a much lower amount of carbohydrates.

This is a general description of what a keto diet does, but that alone is not sufficient to base a decision upon. I know, I was certainly attracted by the general idea and how it sounded, but I needed more than just a line or two about what keto does. I needed to know exactly what goes on within our body and how keto can fit the picture, especially for people who have a few pounds popping out of proportion and age that is rapidly approaching the 60 years mark.

The Science Behind It

The idea behind most diets remains the same. One needs to reduce the amount of carbs intake in a day, and the weight should fall. The problem is that most diets require you to stop eating or skip meals to bring the carb level down. For a very long time, I had wondered if there was any other way to address this issue. Certainly, the idea of losing weight is appealing. It is a motivator that pushes us to stop eating and force our body to start converting stored fats into fuel to burn. Sounds good, but the hunger that comes in is a killer.

The catch behind cutting down on carbs is simple; it makes your body run low on glucose. When that happens, the state of ketosis is in effect. This is where ketones come to the rescue as your body's natural fuel backup. Here's a little fact: we only ever enter into the state of ketosis if we starve ourselves for a few days, not just overnight or by skipping a meal. That, then, is quite a tough prospect.

In keto, things work a little differently, and fortunately, a little more friendly. The principle remains the same, you force your body to switch the ketosis mode on, but instead of starving yourself for food, you just cut down the amount of carbs while continuing to consume other nutrients. Slice it any way you like, but this is genuinely more interesting and easier to do.

By removing all sorts of carbs, including but not limited to complex carbs, starches, and refined carbs, we will force our body to lose glucose and be left with no other source to acquire more. This will then switch our body into ketosis to allow ketones to make their way to the brain and resume normal functions. Our brain requires either glucose or ketones to function, and through ketosis, it gets the necessary supply.

What follows afterwards is a continuous process of our body breaking down fats into ketones regardless of how much protein or fat you consume. The result is a satisfying hunger and weight loss that changes everything for you; a feat many diets cannot deliver.

The world has been taken by storm at just how easy this diet can be and how it can deliver magnificent results. Keto diets are almost for everyone who are suffering from weight issues and are unable to lose their extra pounds. Through careful selection of food and monitoring the intake the keto way, you should be able to see the results rather quickly.

It goes without saying that for a weight loss solution, keto is looking up as a perfect contender. Not only do you not need to give up eating, but you can enjoy scrumptious meals while losing your weight through techniques which otherwise would require you to starve to near death. In addition to these facts, most keto recipes are extremely easy to cook, and most of them taste equally delicious. This means you do not have to rely on bitter-tasting drinks, weird looking food, or lack thereof.

Keto is quite popular, and for a very good reason. It genuinely promotes healthy eating without pushing anyone into a state of jeopardy. The success rate of keto is rather high. While there are no specific numbers to suggest the exact rate, it is only fair to state that those who have the will to change their lifestyle and are okay adjusting to new eating habits, almost every one of them will make it through as a success story.

What is Ketosis?

Ketosis is a metabolic state where the body is efficiently using fat for energy. In a regular diet, carbohydrates produce glucose, which is used to provide energy. Glucose is stored in the body in fat cells that travel via the bloodstream. People gain weight when there is more fat stored than being used as energy.

Glucose is formed through the consumption of sugar and starch—Namely carbohydrates. The sugars may be in the form of natural sugars from fruit or milk, or they may be formed from processed sugar. Starches like pasta, rice or starchy vegetables like potatoes and corn, form glucose as well. The body breaks down the sugars from these foods into glucose. Glucose and insulin combined to help to carry glucose into the bloodstream so the body can use glucose as energy. The glucose that is not used is stored in the liver and muscles

In order for the body to supply ketones for use as fuel, the body must use up all the reserves of glucose. In order to do this, there must be a condition of the body of starvation, low carbohydrates, passing, or strenuous exercise. A very low carb diet, the production of ketones what her to feel the body and brain.

Why Is It Important for People Over 50?

Now comes the interesting part. I am sure you have been wondering how it will help you, a person who is 50 years or more in age, and why is it so important, right? Do not worry as I shall provide you with an answer that satisfies both questions.

A few minutes ago, we read how keto diet pushes our body into ketosis; a state where ketones take over the role of glucose. That may sound good for younger people than you, but the fact is that it is actually a better fit for someone your age. Why, I hear you ask?

As you grow in age, the body's natural fat-burning ability reduces.

When that happens, your body stops receiving a healthy dose of nutrients properly, which is why you will develop diseases and ailments. With the keto diet, you are pushing the body into ketosis and bypassing the need to worry about your body's ability to burn fat. Once in ketosis, your body will now burn fat forcefully for survival.

Once more, your system will now start to regain strength. An even better aspect that follows is your insulin level because it drops. If you are someone diagnosed with diseases such as type 2 diabetes and others, the drop in insulin might even reverse the effects and eliminate the diseases from your body altogether.

There are studies underway, and most of them suggest that the keto diet is far more beneficial to those above 50 than it is for those under this age bracket. A quick search on Google and you are immediately overwhelmed with over 93 million results, most of which explain the benefits of the keto diet for people above 50. That is a staggering number for a diet plan that has only been around a few years.

It is also important to highlight that as we get older, we start losing more than just the ability to burn fat. During this phase of our life, once we hit around 50 years of age, we come across various obstacles, some chronic in nature, which transpire only because our body is no longer able to function at rates like it did when we were young. Ketogenic diets help us regain that edge and feel energized from within.

There are hundreds of thousands of stories, all pointing out how this revolutionary diet is especially helpful for older adults and the elderly. It is, therefore, a no-brainer for people above 50 who have spent ages trying to search for a healthy lifestyle choice of diet. With such a high success rate, there is no harm in trying, right?

Before the keto phenomenon, there was the Atkins diet. The Atkins diet was also a low carb diet, just like its keto counterpart. This form of diet also became a huge hit with the masses. However, unlike keto, the Atkins diet provided weight loss while putting a person through constant hunger. Keto, on the other hand, takes away that element, and it does that using ketosis.

Constant exposure to ketosis reduces appetite, hence taking away the biggest hurdle in most diets. The Atkins diet failed to address that front, which is why it was more of a hit and miss. However, credit where it is due, the Atkins diet did garner quite a bit of fame.

However, since the inception of keto, things have changed dramatically.

A study was conducted where 34 overweight adults were monitored and observed for 12 months. All of them were put on keto diets. The end result showed that participants had lower HgbA1c (hemoglobin A1c) levels, experienced significant weight loss, and were more likely to completely discontinue their medications for diabetes.

All in all, the keto diet is shaping up to be quite a promising candidate for older adults. Not only will this diet allow us to lead a healthier lifestyle, but it will also curb our ailments and ensure high energy around the clock. That is quite the resume for a diet, and one that now seems too attractive to pass up. This is the point where I made up my mind and decided to give the keto diet a go, and I recommend the same to you.

Whether you are a man or a woman, if you have put on weight, or you are suffering from ailments like type 2 diabetes, consider this as your ticket to a care-free world where you will lead a healthy life and rise out of the ailments eventually.

Keto has been producing results which have attracted the top minds and researchers for a fairly long time. Considering the unique nature of this lifestyle of eating, the results have been rather encouraging.

Body Changes after 50

We are all getting older. Of course, you are no exception. This process is inevitable, and it makes your life saturated in all aspects. When you're 50-something, you gain wisdom and life experience, you build meaningful relationships and mental strength. But don't forget that not only internal changes occur after age 50. Your body also changes, and you need to prepare for that.

Your Metabolic Rate Slows Down

When you have reached the age of 50, your body starts digesting food in a different way as a result of a decreased metabolic rate. Chemical reactions inside your body that are responsible for burning the calories you consume become slower. It is entirely normal and doesn't mean that you should eat less or reduce the portion sizes on your plate. This peculiarity implies that you should pay more attention to your meal plan as you age and choose the food that fits best for your nutritional needs as well as goals.

Your Muscle Power Decreases

At the old age, muscle mass and, therefore, strength reduces. Physical inactivity and an unhealthy diet are the leading causes of this negative change in a 50-something-year-old's body. But it is in your power to prevent this change.

Your Bones Become More Brittle

When it comes to the bones, you gotta understand that their condition is also more likely to change after 50. Hormonal imbalance, and loss of calcium and other crucial minerals in bones result in low bone density and a higher risk of injury.

Your Excess Weight Increases

Perhaps the only thing that rises with age is the figure on your scales. As you get older, you can experience disappointing changes in your body. In most cases, you notice them when looking in the mirror and weighing yourself. Extra pounds are a real problem for people who are over 50 and the most unpleasant task is getting rid of this dead weight. Well, this is one more reason why you need to focus on the Keto diet and look closely at all the benefits of this low-carb eating plan for older people.

Benefits of the Keto Diet for People over 50

If you're a person who's already celebrated your 50th birthday, that doesn't mean that your life becomes dull from here on, and you don't know how to spend your free time. Quite the opposite! You may often feel time-crunch because of work, family, and generally because of various life situations. Actually, it can be quite difficult to make time for yourself and, moreover, finding time to plan a healthy diet is more likely to be last on the list of your priorities. However, you can change your attitude towards your nutritional needs and move them to the top of that list when you find out all the benefits of a low-carb, high-fat diet for older people.

- **Improved Physical and Mental Health**

With ageing, you might notice an energy level drop due to different environmental and biological reasons. If you want to feel happy, active, and dynamic, pay closer attention to the Keto diet. Remember, reducing your carbohydrate intake usually leads to increasing your vital forces. When you start consuming a lower number of carbs, the body has to burn more fat to fuel itself. This process causes fat synthesis and ketone production, i.e. breaking down accumulated fat for energy. In such a way, the low-carbohydrate diet can stimulate brainpower and positive changes in cognition (like improving memory and concentration).

- **Faster Metabolism**

Older people have a slower metabolism. But thanks to the Keto diet, this problem can be solved. Excluding carb intake from your diet plan can help you to maintain healthy levels of blood sugar and, as a result, rev up your metabolism.

- **Weight-Shedding**

It is no big secret that as a person gets older, shedding weight gets harder. People after 50 face the challenge of weight-loss for a variety of reasons (from increasing levels of stress, slower metabolic rate to rapid muscle loss). The struggle with excess weight may take a lot of time and effort for people over the age of 50. But there is a way out, and it is called the Keto diet.

This peculiar diet is highly effective for losing weight because it boosts the metabolism of fat, and the body itself starts shedding stored fat. As an added bonus, people who stick to the Keto diet get a reduced appetite, which helps to prevent over-eating and, thus, quicker weight loss. Unlike many low-fat diets, the Ketogenic one doesn't recommend you to track your calories or eat less. There's no need for that! Keto usually leaves you feeling full and satisfied after a meal.

- **Better Sleep**

At an old age, people tend to have trouble sleeping. A lot of people over 50 experience such sleep disorders as insomnia, sleep apnea, restless leg syndrome, and sleepwalking. People aged 50 and over should know that a long-term Ketogenic diet can have a positive impact on sleep. A significant reduction in carb intake and, at the same time, a substantial increase in fat intake create favorable conditions for a night of deeper sleep, eliminate certain sleep disturbance triggers, and make a person more energetic when the sun is up.

- **Protection from Age-Related Diseases**

According to various scientific studies, the Keto diet can reduce the risks for specific age-related diseases, such as diabetes, different kinds of cancer, cardiovascular diseases, mental disorders, Parkinson's Disease, multiple sclerosis, and fatty liver disease.

Chapter 2: Keto for Women Over 50

For married couples looking to improve their lifestyle, continue to read on.

Women—we go through so much in life, don't we? From growing up, discovering the joys of life, pursuing a promising career, becoming a mother; there is so much that changes within such a short span of time.

While that is a part of life, what anyone would genuinely try and avoid would be the part where we put on excessive weight that we carry around like an unneeded luggage. It is embarrassing, it is distracting, and it is causing quite a few internal issues as well.

If you thought the biggest hurdle you will face when you hit 50 is a big belly, think again. This isn't the only problem we face. While there are those who would say that having a generous belly is the biggest problem, I firmly believe that there are more serious issues to worry about than that. When it comes to women, well things aren't looking good.

Our bodies, since birth, continuously undergo changes. Most of these changes do not harm us and are only natural. However, once we enter into our 50s, things are a lot different. Now, any changes within our body will directly affect how we perform, operate and work. If we were to keep these changes unchecked and pay no close attention, things would take a turn for the worse.

Most of these issues will remain the same for men as well; however, due to the chemistry of our bodies and differences, both internal and external, both would end up facing a variety of issues exclusive to their gender.

There are a few ways we can avoid these issues. Some of these ways require you to go back in time and start working out from a very young age, control your diet, and change your habits. Obviously, that is the stuff of science fiction and hence is out of the equation.

Other ways would include visiting a doctor and getting pills and energy boosters to help us feel better while taking more pills to fight off diabetes, high blood pressure, and other health issues. This way is not just hectic but far too complicated as well.

For a very long time, the only other way was to avoid worrying too much and hope that life would fix issues itself, and that never ended well for many. People were then left with a worry and a gap that nothing was able to fill. In comes ketogenic diet.

Call it a need of the hour, a savior in disguise or anything you like, the fact remains that this is proving to be a popular option that is not only delivering results but is also helping millions to maintain a healthy lifestyle and reverse some of the damage their bodies have suffered.

Numerous studies have gone on to support the idea that keto diets are far more effective for the older men and women compared to the younger folks. With so much to look forward to and so little to sacrifice, it does make sense to state that keto is essentially becoming your permanent way of life once you hit 50, but why is that? Why is it that me and so many others are proclaiming keto as an important lifestyle choice for women above 50? The answer to this involves some explanation, but I will do my best to do just that!

Keto: The Need of the Hour

Calling something the need of the hour is quite a statement. Anyone to claim something being so important must have sufficient material and facts to back such a claim with. While I have provided what exactly keto does, there is much to be learned and explored of just why keto is important for women over the age of 50.

So far, we have learned that women over 50 would face issues like:

- Being overweight
- Running low on energy
- Feeling drowsy and lethargic all the time
- Unable to focus on a task
- Glucose levels going haywire
- Blood pressure issues

These are the most common ones but dig a little deeper and you quickly realize that these are just the tip of the iceberg that lies hidden in plain sight.

Menopause

There comes an age in a woman's life where her menstrual cycle will finally end. This is a phase that means your ovaries stop releasing eggs, better known as ovulation, and therefore menstruation ends. This condition is generally observed in women above the age of 40. There is no defined age that shows when a woman can expect menopause.

There are times where women may experience menopause prematurely as well. This happens if a woman has undergone surgeries like hysterectomy (surgery that involves removal of ovaries). It can also happen from any injuries that may have caused damage to the ovaries. If this happens before the age of 40, it is classified as premature menopause.

Menopause, as harmless as it sounds, can be quite a troubling phase for women. The hot flashes you experience will keep you up at night, with an elevated heartbeat. The constant feeling of being irritated and a clear downfall in your sex life can contribute greatly towards you feeling more and more grumpy.

Menopause takes a toll on your hormonal balance and the newly developed imbalance then pushes your body to gain massive weight, experience mood swings like never before and a libido that is crashing faster than you can imagine.

If you think this is bad, here are some other issues that menopause can lead to:

- Chronic stress

- Anxiety

- Insulin spike

- Type 2 Diabetes

- Heart Diseases

- Polycystic ovary syndrome (PCOS)

The overall picture, then, is grim! Fortunately, a difference of lifestyle and a carefully thought-out diet plan can change all that for you. I am not saying it happens overnight or within a week, but the profound impacts are felt rather quick. In the longer run, keto will rescue you and your body from impending doom and allow you to lead a life without worrying about keeping a glucose monitor or any of the typical health-related equipment near you.

The keto diet, while there are many classes of it, helps your hormones to remain in shape and balanced. This means that you do not have to worry about the insulin or any other hormones, hence minimizing the hot flashes and other symptoms. Even if they occur, they will be minor and far less painful.

Moreover, the keto diet jump-starts your sex drive. The fat-rich diet improves fat-soluble vitamin absorption. Not to forget it especially helps with vitamin D, a vital piece that goes missing with age. All in all, this provides all the drive you need to have intimate moments even in your fifties.

Heart Diseases

Keto diets help women over 50 to shed those extra pounds. Reducing any amount of weight greatly reduces the chances of a heart attack or any other heart complications. Through the carefully selected diet routine, not only are you losing weight and enjoying scrumptious meals, but you are significantly boosting your heart's health and reviving yourself from the otherwise dull state that you may have been in before.

Diabetes Control

Needless to say, the careful selection of ingredients, when cooked together, provide rich nutrients, free from any processed or harmful contents such as sugar. Add to that the fact that keto automatically controls your insulin levels. The result is a glucose level that is always under control, and continued control would lead to a day where you will say goodbye to the medications you might be taking for diabetes.

And so Much More!

By taking up the challenge and adapting the keto way, you are ensuring yourself one of the safest journeys into the older years, if not the safest of the lot. Sure, there will be days where you may miss a food or two, but that craving will be overshadowed by the benefits the keto diet will bring for you.

With the help of the keto diet, you can expect a few more benefits, such as:

- Improved and stable blood pressure levels

- A deeper sleep for those suffering from insomnia

- Improved kidney function

- More energy that lasts all-day

- Improved bodily functions

All Set to Begin?

Great! Let me be the first one to let you know that you are not too late to start. The fact is, no one is ever too late to change their eating, sleeping, and working habits. All it takes is a spark of motivation, and if you are reading this line, you already have that spark. All you need now is to grab a pen and a paper to note down some fine recipes and jot down the things you need and the things you should avoid. Better yet, maintain a little diary or a notebook which you can refer to whenever you wish.

Chapter 3: Keto for Men Over 50

Men—much like us women, you also go through quite a lot of internal and external changes. These include but are not limited to physical changes, habitual changes, and so on. While the chemistry inside the body of both remains broadly the same, whether young or old, there are things which men are more likely to develop or lose than women. These include some diseases, ailments, infections, habitual changes, and disorders. The worst news is; it happens as soon as you cross 45 years of age. That means you are at least five years late already, or at least that is what you think.

I was discussing about how a woman experiences changes within herself once she is 50 and up, I mentioned that it is never too late to begin your journey and pick up your very first keto routine. All it takes is a mind that is poised, a will that is evident, and a clear goal in sight. That is quite literally it.

However, unlike most diets which you can begin right away, there are a few things I should point out which men should keep an eye out for. Consider these as soft reminders or suggestions before you take up the keto challenge.

Keto diet is a lifestyle: Keto it is not a diet that you do just for two weeks, and then resume your normal food and carb intake. This is a proper lifestyle that you will need to adopt and live with. As long as you continue abiding by its rules, you will continue to enjoy the benefits it has to offer.

- **Keto is not only meant for women**: There are those who actually believe that keto was designed specifically for women. I am here to set things right and let you know that keto is for both men and women.

- **Keto does not require you to cut down on your eating habits**: Not at all. With that said though, it does make you modify those habits by changing what you consume instead of how much you consume.

- **Keto food items may pose a risk to people with special medical conditions**: It is something that most websites, blogs, and articles fail to mention. If you suffer from issues like high cholesterol, be sure to do a bit of research regarding what you can use instead of a specific ingredient.

With that said, let us get down to details and find out just why keto is so important for men who are 50 years old and above.

50 Marks the Start of Troubles

Well, in all fairness, troubles for men may start a little sooner than that, but the reason I said that is because some of these troubles, such as diseases or issues related to obesity and weight gain, take some time to manifest themselves. It is usually around the 50-year mark where these issues come up almost immediately.

Now that you are within this age group, and are nearing your retirement age, there are so many things which can cause you to lose your patience, your focus, and depreciate your health as well. The biggest of these would be stress; the stress of not knowing what you will do once you have retired.

This stress can cause you to have insomnia, a massive eating disorder, and ultimately a body that is quickly running out of shape. With each passing year, you are incurring extra expenses upon yourself and trying to find a shirt and trousers that fits your new size. I completely understand that none of us, men or women, like to see that.

Stress is just the start of things; I haven't even begun to point out the medical issues a man's body can develop and be bombarded with. To give you an idea of what a 50-year-old male faces who is not observing any kind of diet, here is a list to digest:

- Anxiety

- Depression

- Uncontrollable blood pressure levels

- Diminishing sex drive

- Increased laziness

- Lack of energy

- Fluctuating insulin levels

Think about it, do any of these really sound the sort of issues you would be okay to face in such an age? Certainly, you need some form of assistance that can help you boost your morale, your spirits, and allow you to control life the way you had always done so.

"Exercise is the answer!" Well, yes and no.

You see, while exercise provides you with the muscular strength and some really good benefits, it is still not the ideal way to cut down on those extra pounds, nor will it allow you to control other bodily disorders. All exercise can do is to keep your body in shape physically. That is all there is to it. There is a simple reason for that.

Exercises are designed to utilize your body's energy and use it to carry out difficult tasks which, as a result, promote more strength and growth of muscles and mass. The keyword to focus here is "energy" and that is exactly where a diet comes in. In this case, we will be focusing on possibly the best diet of them all: keto.

The good news is that by combining your love of keto and exercise, you end up with the perfect duo that is always ready to complement each other. While they do that, you, the actual end-user, gets to enjoy a perfectly healthy lifestyle that is free from any harmful carbs or other nutrients.

For men over the age of 50, it is very much important to remain in good shape. This is something you would want to do as it allows you to carry out more tasks relatively easy and keeps you active throughout the day. But wait, there is more to keto than just that.

Helping You Live Longer

Through adopting a keto diet plan for your meals, and adding exercise to that, you are most likely to lead a longer life. Why do I say this? If you haven't noticed already, the keto diet comes with quite a lot of benefits.

The keto diet helps you to improve your blood sugar levels. This eliminates quite a lot of issues, such as type 2 diabetes. Additionally, the keto plan helps you in keeping carbs at bay. This, in return pushes your body to absorb fats as fuel instead. By doing so, your body will start to burn fats quicker than usual, and that is some good news for everyone.

As you grow old, some functions fade out while others slow down to a snail's pace. An example of the latter is the rate at which our body burns fat now versus how it used to burn fat when you were younger. There is a significant difference, and with keto you can recover that ability fairly easy as it trains your body to switch into ketosis mode.

This new change within your body would then make room for more energy. The more energy you have, the better you can work, focus, and carry out tasks. Finally, the keto diet never asks you to stop eating, and that means you always have a healthy meal waiting for you at least three times a day, if not more.

Combine all that and your body automatically starts to feel fresher and healthier. This will also have a drastic effect on your personality. With more confidence, you will be able to deal with the public and lead a happier life.

Good Under the Sheets

Let's be honest; we all have a few things on our priority list which we cannot compromise on. One of them is sharing those intimate moments with our partner, right? The bad part is the libido, the thing that makes this magic possible, starts to drop low as we approach the half-century mark. Once we cross that, the fall increases drastically, and we feel the lack of urge for intimacy and a lower sex drive.

When something as important and pleasurable as sex dies out, life takes a toll. Without it, both men and women grow grumpy, irritated and lose their charm. While women have to worry about the menopause issues, men get to deal with things like erectile dysfunction. In either case, it is the stuff of nightmares.

With the help of keto though, things can change and change for the better. With a selection of some fine ingredients, you can cook up some food that will top your body up with the energy, strength, and the libido that you need to get back in action. Add to that a few exercises, and you would be as fit as you were quite a few years younger. Relive the moments with your loved ones and rekindle the fire that seemingly went out for good.

Strengthening the Bones

One of the biggest issues' men face when they cross the magical number of 50 is the rapidly deteriorating strength within their bones. While they may have been able to walk for miles without breaking a sweat, back in the day, they would now face an incredibly tough time climbing a set of stairs no more than two stories high. This is an alarming situation, and one that needs a solution ASAP!

Fortunately, the keto diet provides some relief to the people suffering from joint aches from osteoarthritis and weakened muscles. Through this diet, the necessary nutrients are released into the body which will then cause a sudden spike within the body, brimming it with energy to carry out tasks that would otherwise seem impossible to do at such an age.

Imagine the keto diet as spinach for Popeye. The minute he eats it, he's all muscles. I should also point out that this is just a reference and that keto does not provide you with such quick results.

Keto Helps to Prevent Certain Cancers

Cancer, whatever the type, is one of the most horrific diseases in existence. Just the mere mention of the word and everyone will immediately be stunned.

Cancers take time to manifest and are usually caused by long prevailing, underlying causes. They do not appear randomly and require the right kind of environment to develop. However, once they appear, time is of the essence. Be late and it is curtains for good.

With the introduction of keto, which was initially introduced within children to control epilepsy, things looked promising. While keto does not prevent all cancers, it is mighty effective against some types of cancers. Some reports have shown significant revival of patients who were aged 50 and above, which provides all the more reason for men above 50 to start on ketogenic diets, if they haven't already done so. Simply put, keto is possibly the only lifestyle men should seek to ensure a healthier life leading into retirement.

Some Side Effects You Should Know

Some of these side effects are universal, meaning that both men and women would face these. However, there are varying studies which suggest some symptoms or side-effects are more prominent within men above 50 as compared to women above 50. Nonetheless, it is a good idea to know what exactly you are dealing with and what you can expect to face as time goes by.

Most of these symptoms will fade away with time, but some may linger on. There is no such symptom that may pose a threat to you or anyone else. However, it is generally a good idea to be prepared to face these as they come. A prepared mind stands a better chance at dealing with things.

The side effects include:

- The dreaded keto flu: A flu-like illness that hits you right in the starting few weeks. Nothing to be alarmed about as this is only because your body is coping with the new changes.

- Keto breath: I do wish this was not the case, but since it exists, it is best to know of it beforehand. Keto breath is quite strong as it contains acetone.

- Tougher visits to the bathroom: You can either develop diarrhea or nasty constipation. However, rest assured, this is a short-term symptom and will go away shortly.

- A massive thirst: Yes! You will feel thirsty quite a lot. It is advisable that you drink plenty of water to ensure you do not suffer worse side-effects because of the added thirst.

As I mentioned, some of these symptoms may be more noticeable for men than women. However, the difference is marginal at best.

I had already warned the ladies to exercise caution before moving on and ensure that they check their conditions first and figure out if they have any special diet needs. Similarly, if men who are 50 and above face any issues, I recommend that you find out what you can eat and what you can't. You can consult a dietician or a doctor and get some details about what is good for you and what isn't. Once that is sorted, all you need is a pen and a notebook to start taking notes.

You will be spending a lot of time in the kitchen, so it is probably a good idea to hone in on your cooking skills. You will need them quite a lot if you truly wish to take benefits from the keto diet.

Chapter 4: Keto for Women vs. Men

In reality, since women and men have been created differently, our approach to Keto Diet may differ and should be different. These are the biological indifferences that we have no control with. We are going to be talking about the differences between males and females when it comes to approaching the Keto Diet.

So how should men do it or women do it? Here's a thing we need to understand about the Keto Diet first and foremost is that it is very bio-individual so that even among men, there are different ways to do it and among women there are different ways as well. So just understand that it is individual and it might take some tweaking as you go throughout the process. But for all men and for all women, it's really important to become Keto adaptive first before we start tweaking things so what we mean by that is you need to do Keto strict for the first thirty days or so until you get adapted. Your body is becoming more efficient, and it is adapting to this new fuel source called ketones and it is going to take a while before your body gets adapted. But once you get adapted here is where there might be some difference in men versus women so some women tend not to do well over the long term with intermittent fasting.

So intermittent fasting is very popular that a lot of people that do Keto do intermittent fasting as well because it puts you in a modified or a modified state of Ketosis so you are making some ketones but women over the long term because of their hormones being different with men and their cycles during that time of the month. They might need to increase their carbohydrate intakes the week before their cycle starts.

So what we recommend to all women out there is that if you have become adapted to the Ketogenic Diet is that you should be cycling in and out of Ketosis from time to time and specifically try it out adding in healthy carbs, not talking about pizza, french fries or soda but healthy carbs like fruit, potatoes, sweet potatoes, maybe a little bit of rice the week before your cycle. Adding those carbohydrates during night time could help out balance those hormones for you so that you don't experience there's side effects from going Keto long term. And that is what we've seen help a lot of women that are clients is adding those in plus you are not as grumpy or angry. This stuff can definitely help out with those symptoms and side effects. So add in carbohydrates the week before your cycle.

For men also, it is best recommended that you test your hormones and get your blood work done every couple of months, so you know how your body is changing and adapting so you know maybe you need to switch things up or maybe do the target a ketogenic diet for a week or two and see how your body responds and adapts. You need to become your own experimentations, so you know what is best for you moving forward.

The truth is, there is a wide variety of people who can benefit from the Ketogenic Diet, whether they are young, old, man, or woman, but the Ketogenic Diet has been known to be especially beneficial for women due to their different hormones and conditions. This diet can be especially beneficial for women who are:

- Lacking results on other diets

- Binge on carbohydrates

- Planning on getting pregnant

- Want a healthy pregnancy

- Struggling with irregular periods

- Struggling with sex hormones

- Going through menopause

When you first begin the Ketogenic Diet, you are most likely anticipating all of the benefits people mention. While those changes will come at some point, you should be aware of the dreaded Keto Flu. Unfortunately, many people do not anticipate for this metabolic change, and they are unable to push through the potential side effects.

With that in mind, you will want to remember that the Keto flu is only going to be temporary! The flu is most prevalent when the body is attempting to transition into the new, ketogenic state. As soon as your body learns how to be fat-adapted, the symptoms will disappear before you know it!

Why Keto for 50+?

As we age, we naturally look for ways to hold onto our youth and energy. It's not uncommon to think about things that promote anti-ageing. Products and lifestyle changes are advertised everywhere, and they are designed to catch your attention, as you grapple with the reality of what it means to be a 50+-year-old woman in our society. Even if you aren't eating for the purposes of anti-aging yet, you have likely thought about it in terms of the way you treat your skin and hair, for example. The great thing about the Keto diet is that it supports maximum health, from the inside out; working hard to make sure that you are in the best shape that you can be in.

For instance, indigestion becomes as common as you age. This happens because the body is not able to break down certain foods as well as it used to. With all of the additives and fillers, we all become used to putting our bodies through discomfort in an attempt to digest regular meals. You are probably not even aware that you are doing this to your body, but upon trying a Keto diet, you will realize how your digestion will begin to change. You will no longer feel bloated or uncomfortable after you eat. If you notice this as a common feeling, you are likely not eating food that is nutritious enough to satisfy your needs and is only resulting in excess calories.

Keto fills you up in all of the ways that you need, allowing your body to truly digest and metabolize all of the nutrients. When you eat your meals, you should not feel the need to overeat in order to overcompensate for not having enough nutrients. Anything that takes stress off of any system in your body is going to become a form of anti-aging. You will quickly find this benefit once you start your Keto journey, as it is one of the first-reported changes that most participants notice. In addition to a healthier digestive system, you will also experience more regular bathroom usage, with little to none of the problems often associated with age.

While weight loss is one of the more common desires for most 50+ women who start a diet plan, the way that the weight is lost matters. If you have ever shed a lot of weight before, you have probably experienced the adverse effects of sagging or drooping skin that you were left to deal with. Keto actually rejuvenates the elasticity in your skin. This means that you will be able to lose weight and your skin will be able to catch up. Instead of having to do copious amounts of exercise to firm up your skin, it should already be becoming firmer each day that you are on the Keto diet. This is something that a lot of participants are pleasantly surprised to find out.

Women also commonly report a natural reduction in wrinkles, and healthier skin and hair growth, in general. Many women who start the diet report that they actually notice reverse effects in their ageing process. While the skin becomes healthier and suppler, it also becomes firmer. Even if you aren't presently losing weight, you will still be able to appreciate the effects that Keto brings to your skin and face. Because your internal systems are becoming healthier by the day, this tends to show on the outside in a short amount of time. You will also begin to feel healthier. While it is possible to read about the experiences of others, there is nothing like feeling this for yourself when you begin Keto.

Everyone, especially women over 50, has day-to-day tasks that are draining and require certain amounts of energy to complete. Ageing can, unfortunately, take away from your energy reserve, even if you get enough sleep at night. It limits the way that you have to live your life, and this can become a very frustrating realization. Most diet plans bring about a sluggish feeling that you are simply supposed to get used to, for example. But Keto does the exact opposite. When you change your eating habits to fit the Keto guidelines, you are going to be hit with a boost of energy. Since your body is truly getting everything that it needs nutritionally, it will repay you with a sustained energy supply. Another common complaint for women over 50 is that, seemingly overnight, your blood sugar levels are going to be more sensitive than usual. While it is important that everyone keeps an eye on these levels, it is especially important for those who are in their 50s and beyond. High blood sugar can be an indication that diabetes is on the way, but Keto can become a preventative measure, that we've already talked about. Additionally, naturally regulating elevated blood sugar levels, also reduces systemic inflammation, which is also common for women over 50. By balancing the immune system, of which inflammation is a part of, common aches and pains are reduced. If, for example, you've noticed that you have been feeling stiff lately, even despite your efforts to exercise and stretching, this is likely due to a normal case of inflamed joints. Inflammation can also affect vital organs and is a precursor to cancer. Keto will support your path to an anti-inflammatory lifestyle.

Sugar is never great for us, but it turns out that sugar can become especially dangerous as we age. What is known as a "sugar sag" can occur when you get older because the excess sugar molecules will attach themselves to skin and protein in your body. This doesn't even necessarily happen because you are eating too much sugar. Average levels of sugar intake can also lead to this sagging as the sugar weakens the strength of your proteins that are supposed to hold you together. With sagging comes even more wrinkles and arterial stiffening.

If you have any anti-ageing concerns, the Keto diet will likely be able to address your worries. It is a diet that works extremely hard while allowing you a fairly simple and direct guideline to follow in return. While your motivation is necessary in order to form a successful relationship with Keto, you won't need to worry about doing anything "wrong" or accidentally breaking from your diet. As long as you know how to give up your sugary foods and drinks while making sure that you are consuming the correct amount of carbs, you will be able to find your own success while on the diet.

As a woman over 50, you'll find that you will feel better, healthier and younger, by implementing the simple steps that will tune your body into processing excess fats for energy. You'll build muscle, lose fat, and look and feel younger. As we've touched on, a Keto diet helps balance your hormones, reversing and/or eliminating many common menopausal signs and symptoms.

Chapter 5: What Is the Keto Flu?

As you probably could have already guessed, the Keto flu is fairly related to the regular flu. The Keto flu comes about because your metabolism is trying to adjust to running on your new form of energy, fat. This is going to be a drastic change for your body, especially because, for the majority of your life, it has been running off glucose or carbohydrates for energy!

When you begin reducing your carb intake, this is going to begin depleting the glucose stores in your body. This switch can be tough on your body, and from here, you will start to experience the flu-like symptoms. If you have ever had the flu before, you already know that it is not a great feeling.

Signs & Symptoms of the Keto Flu

So, what can you expect from this infamous Keto Flu? Some of the more common symptoms include:

- Low Energy Levels
- Sugar Cravings
- Lack of Focus
- Inability to Concentrate
- Irritability
- Heart Palpitations

- Insomnia
- Muscle Cramps
- Muscle Soreness
- Constipation
- Diarrhea
- Confusion
- Dizziness
- Nausea
- Stomach Pain
- Overall Brain Fog

If you are starting the Ketogenic Diet for the first time and are nervously awaiting the Keto-Flu, the symptoms listed above will generally start up around the first day or two of your diet. It should be noted that the length and strength of the symptoms are going to vary depending on the person. In fact, some people are lucky enough to skip the Keto flu altogether! Either way, you can rest assured that the symptoms will only last two weeks, at most. The sooner your body becomes fat-adapted, the better you will feel.

Causes of the Keto Flu

As you expand your knowledge of the Ketogenic Diet, you should be aware that there are four main causes of the keto flu. We will go over each source in detail below to help you lessen the blow of the flu in the first place.

Keto Adaption

Keto adaption is going to be one of the main culprits behind the Keto Flu. The body is incredibly complex and has two primary processes for energy. This includes glycolysis, which is burning glucose for energy and beta-oxidation, which is burning fat for energy. As your body adjusts, you will be switching from one process to the other. This switch is called your metabolic flexibility.

What many people don't realize is that genetics play a major role in our metabolic flexibility. If your metabolic flexibility is low, you are more likely to experience the symptoms of the keto flu. For this reason, some people handle the energy switch easier than others.

Carbohydrate Withdrawal

When you first make the switch to the Ketogenic Diet, you can expect a number of symptoms like cravings for sugar, irritability, and mood swings. There are studies that suggest that our brain is affected by sugar, similar to the way that it is affected by drugs such as cocaine or heroin. When we eat sugar, it releases the "feel good," hormone, dopamine. If you are not getting your "fix," your body is going to protest.

For this reason, when you begin to reduce the number of carbs in your diet, you can expect some of these symptoms. If your diet is currently heavy in refined carbs, sugars, and processed foods, you may have it worse off than others. While this doesn't mean you should jump off the Keto wagon instantly, you should anticipate the flu before it happens.

Lack of Micronutrients

People who first begin the Ketogenic Diet may have a hard time finding the proper balance when it comes to their macronutrients and their micronutrients. I understand that it is difficult enough learning what you can and cannot eat, but these micronutrients are going to be important when it comes to your health.

As you begin the Ketogenic Diet, you already know that you are going to be cutting out a large number of grains, fruits, and vegetables. In order to make up for this, you will need to make sure you are eating a proper amount of keto-friendly foods that will still help you get your micronutrients in. Some of the best foods you can incorporate will be:

- Olive Oil
- Coconut Butter
- Fatty-cut Meat
- Seeds
- Nuts
- Fish
- Asparagus
- Spinach
- Eggplant
- Full-fat dairy

If you find yourself unable to get your micronutrients in, you may want to consider a supplement. Whether it is a multivitamin or a micronutrient powder, you will want to make sure that the item is free from additives, fillers, and sugars. This way, you won't have to worry about non-keto ingredients kicking you out of ketosis.

Electrolyte Imbalance

Last, but definitely not least, we have the electrolyte imbalance. When you begin to make the change of decreasing the number of high carb foods in your diet, you can expect your body to begin losing water at an extremely fast pace.

This happens because the glucose that is stored in your body is bound to anywhere from 2-3 grams of water. As your body begins to adapt, your cells are going to use up the stored glycogen, meaning that the water weight you have been holding onto is going to get flushed out.

When all of this water is flushed out of your system, it is easy to become dehydrated and suffer from an imbalance of electrolytes. Once you become dehydrated, you may experience normal symptoms such as fatigue, headaches, and muscle pain. You will continue to feel this way until you balance your system out again.

For this reason, it will be vital that you are replacing the water and minerals that you are losing during this adaption period. The important minerals you will want to consider including potassium, magnesium, and sodium. By increasing your intake of these minerals, it can help ease your transition period.

The good news is that you will not feel like this forever! These symptoms are only temporary and will reduce as you learn how to put your body into ketosis properly. The even better news is that you can help get rid of the keto flu faster than you thought! Below, you will find some of my favorite tips and tricks of getting rid of the keto flu and jumping into the benefits of the Ketogenic Diet.

How to Get Over the Keto Flu

The anticipation of getting the keto flu can seem overwhelming, but the good news is that you are going to be able to help yourself. The reason people suffer from the keto flu for so long is that they have no idea what is happening to their body! Most people assume that they have to deal with the bad symptoms to get to the benefits of the diet. The truth is, these signs and symptoms from your body are like a cry for help! You don't just feel like junk for no reason! You will want to take the time to listen to your body and see how you can help yourself.

With that in mind, there are several steps you can take to help get you through the keto flu. Below, you will find some of my best tips to help you get over the keto flu and into ketosis with as little misery as possible.

Drink Up and Stay Hydrated

The number one tip I can give you as you begin the ketogenic diet is to stay hydrated! Even if you think that you are drinking enough water, you probably aren't. Staying hydrated should be your top priority as you begin the transition period into ketosis.

As mentioned, water loss is to be expected as you begin your new diet, so these liquids need to be replenished simultaneously. The more often you are drinking, the easier the transition will come. You will see how much drinking water is going to reduce those awful symptoms of nausea, fatigue, and even those wicked headaches.

The best trick up my sleeve to help you drink more water through the day is to keep it in sight! I have a reusable water bottle that is by my side all day long. If you have a visual cue, it acts as an instant reminder to drink more water. I also suggest drinking a majority of the water during the day because it isn't so fun getting up to use the bathroom ten times a night.

Think Electrolytes

While we are on the topic of getting enough water, you will want to keep in mind that balancing your electrolytes is going to be just as important.

Before the ketogenic diet, many people don't have to worry about their electrolytes unless they are highly athletic. As mentioned, your body is about to flush a mass majority of your water weight and electrolytes out of your system during this transition period. With that in mind, it should be noted that people lose electrolytes differently. The good news is that there are several ways for you to mitigate this imbalance.

The first tip I have for you will be increasing your sodium intake! When you increase the sodium in your diet, this could help counterbalance the water loss that is happening in your body. With that in mind, you will want to consider a supplement of Himalayan pink salt rather than the table salt most people have in their house. You would be amazed at the additives found in simple table salt!

Next, you will want to consider eating keto-friendly foods that are rich in potassium. Potassium is in charge of energy production, body temperature, bladder control, heartbeat regulation, and even muscle cramping. If you find yourself having symptoms in any of these areas, you probably need to up your potassium levels. Some of the best sources of this will be pumpkin seeds, mushrooms, and delicious avocado!

Another mineral you will want to make sure you are getting is magnesium. When people have low magnesium levels, this could lead to insulin resistance and depression. To ensure you are getting enough of this micronutrient in your diet, you will want to include food sources like dark chocolate, macadamia nuts, pumpkin seeds, and salmon.

On the Ketogenic Diet, calcium is also going to be important. While most people think that calcium is only important for bone health, it is also vital for your cardiovascular health, muscle contractions, and blood clotting. For this reason, it is a good idea to consume calcium-rich foods like salmon, chia seeds, and leafy greens.

Increase Fats

When your body begins switching over to its new source of energy, you are going to want to make sure that you are providing it with enough fat! Unfortunately, many people are shy about their fat intake when they are first starting their diet because we have been told our whole life that fat is bad! Now that your body is no longer using carbohydrates and sugar as energy, you will need to give your body what it needs!

As you increase your fat consumption while reducing your carb consumption, this will help push your body into using the fat as energy. If you need, you can always supplement with MCT oil to help increase your ketone levels. It is also a good idea to up your fat source and includes foods such as:

- Coconut Oil
- Cacao Butter
- Olive Oil
- Heavy Cream
- Ghee
- Grass-fed Butter
- Avocado Oil
- Bacon Fat
- Walnuts
- Chia Seeds
- Pecans
- Flaxseed

- Fatty Fish

- Sesame Seeds

Work it Out

The next way to help get you over the keto flu will be exercise! This can be hard for some people, especially if they are unable to work through the symptoms provided by the keto flu in the first place. For this reason, I highly suggest light exercise anywhere from two to three times a week.

As you begin moving your body, this will help the switch drastically. As soon as you get over the keto flu, you will be able to resume your normal exercise routine. If you are first starting out, I highly suggest low-intensity exercises. You can try something like yoga, swimming, or even a light walk. With exercise, you will be able to boost your metabolic flexibility and get over the keto flu before you even know it.

Preventing the Keto Flu

While it is beneficial knowing how to get over the keto flu, it is even better knowing how you can prevent it in the first place! If you are like everyone else in the world, you simply do not have the time to get sick! The good news is that there are some ways that you may be able to skip the keto flu altogether.

Follow the Diet

One of the main reasons beginners fall into the Keto-Flu is due to the fact that they are not following the diet the way they are supposed to! The keto diet best when you are getting the proper micronutrients as well as the right number of macronutrients.

The key to getting to your results is learning how to balance your nutritional needs. Yes, you could hit your macronutrients eating nothing but cottage cheese, but this is a sure way to dive right into the Keto flu. While it is going to be important for you to avoid carbohydrates, you will want to learn how to incorporate plenty of vegetables and seeds to help you get the nutrients you need.

The Power of Sleep

Unfortunately, many people are unaware of how important sleep is for the body. When you are first starting the Ketogenic diet, you will want to get at least seven to eight hours of sleep at night. When you are sleeping more, this could help reduce the fatigue and stress that comes along with the metabolism switch. If you struggle with sleep at night, you may want to consider a couple of power naps during the day!

Supplement

If you feel nothing is working, you can always consider taking a supplement or two. While, of course, you can get everything you need from a balanced diet, some people prefer the ease of a supplement.

Chapter 6: Health Benefits of the Ketogenic Diet

As you can tell, there are some extremely complex biological processes behind the Ketogenic Diet. When you first start this diet out, you will want to consult with a doctor before you begin any changes. As far as any diet goes, it is crucial that you choose one that is going to benefit you rather than do more harm. For this reason, be sure to consult with a professional before you experiment on yourself.

With that in mind, why begin any diet if it isn't going to benefit you? Before you dive into the diet itself, let's learn all of the incredible ways that the Ketogenic Diet can help you. Whether you are looking to lose weight, gain energy, or improve brain function, the ketogenic diet may be just what you were searching for.

Brain Benefits

As you begin to change the fuel source for your body, this includes significant fuel sources for your brain as well. Studies have found that through the Ketogenic Diet, individuals were able to increase the stability of their neurons as well as the up-regulation of the mitochondrial enzymes and brain mitochondria.

With that in mind, scientists have been studying how a Ketogenic Diet may be able to benefit those who have Alzheimer's disease. It seems as though through diet, individuals have been able to enhance their memory as well as increase cognition. When this happens, a diet may be able to bring improvement to individuals with all different stages of dementia.

For those who do not need to worry about Parkinson's disease or Alzheimer's disease, the Ketogenic Diet is also beneficial in increasing mental focus, clarity. It could potentially grant less frequent and less intense migraines. Generally, these conditions are related to altered brain chemistry and stable blood sugar levels, both helped by the Ketogenic Diet.

Heart Disease

Another major benefit that makes people take a look at the Ketogenic Diet is the downstream effects of the diet on blood glucose levels. As you begin to cut carbohydrates from your diet, it can help keep your blood glucose stable and low. By doing this, individuals have been able to keep their blood pressure in check and are also able to lower their triglyceride levels.

When people first begin a Ketogenic Diet, they feel that it is counterintuitive to eat a higher percentage of fat in order to lower the triglycerides, but the truth is, fat has had a bad rep this whole time! In fact, it is eating excessive carbohydrates, especially fructose, that is the culprit behind increasing triglycerides! The truth is, through this new diet, you will be able to raise your good cholesterol and lower your bad cholesterol.

Fight Cancer

When it comes to cancer, it is essential that you seek medical attention before you try to take your life into your own hands through diet. It is highly advised that you listen to your doctor's advice when it comes down to cancer treatment. However, there have been articles published based around cancer and the ketogenic diet.

In 2014, Dom D'Agostino's lab published an article based around ketones being able to decrease tumor cell viability in mice that had metastatic cancer. Within this article, it was found that, generally, cancer cells will express an abnormal metabolism that is characterized when glucose consumption is increased. When this happens, the genes begin to mutate, and the mitochondrial begins to malfunction. In the studies, it is found that cancer cells are unable to use ketone bodies as energy, therefore inhibiting the viability of the tumor cell in the first place!

Improve Sleep and Energy Levels

Unfortunately, many individuals underestimate how important sleep is. The good news is that after only four or five days on the ketogenic diet, many individuals have reported that they already begin to benefit from higher energy levels. On a scientific level, this may be due to the fact that through your new ketogenic diet, you will be stabilizing your insulin levels. As your body becomes stabilized, this will help provide you with a ready source of energy rather than experiencing the spikes and crashes.

As far as sleeping goes, the ketogenic diet affects sleep are still being studied. Right now, it seems as though through diet, individuals are able to decrease the time they spend in REM and increase slow-wave sleep patterns. It is believed that this is due to a biochemical shift in the brain as your body learned to use ketones as energy. Either way, you will be sleeping more in-depth and longer than before, granting you a fresh start to each day!

Decrease Inflammation

Inflammation is a strange defense mechanism used in the body to help the immune system recognize any damaged cells, pathogens, or irritants. Through inflammation, the body is able to identify these issues and begin the healing process. While this is beneficial for the most part, it, unfortunately, can persist longer than needed and will end up causing more harm than good.

If you have inflammation in your body, you may experience symptoms such as pain, redness, swelling, immobility, and sometimes even heat. But, these signs only apply to the inflammations on the skin. Sometimes, inflammation can happen within our internal organs, and that is when we experience symptoms such as fever, abdominal pain, chest pain, mouth sores, and even fatigue.

Studies have found that the key player in inflammation, and the diseases associated with it, is suppressed BHB. Luckily through the ketogenic diet, BHB is one of the primary ketones you will be producing as you begin your new diet. This meaning that you will be able to help issues, including IBS, eczema, psoriasis, acne, and even arthritis, all through diet!

Gastrointestinal and Gallbladder Health

If you suffer from heartburn or acid reflux on a daily basis, you may want to take a good, hard look at your diet. Unfortunately, many sugary foods, nightshade vegetables, and grain-based foods are major culprits of both heartburn and acid reflux. With that in mind, it shouldn't come as a surprise that when you change your diet to include low-carb foods, these symptoms will disappear almost instantly. The reason you experience these issues is through an autoimmune response, bacterial issue, and inflammation caused by these foods in the first place.

Another benefit of the Ketogenic Diet will be the altering of the microbiome found in your gut. An individual known as Dr. Eric Westman found that through diet, individuals are able to significantly reduce health issues as they change their microbiome. In fact, he believes that when you take away carbohydrates, this can fix just about any gastrointestinal issues that affect a number of different people.

Along those same lines, research has also found that carbohydrates may be a significant culprit behind gallstones as well. As far as the Ketogenic Diet goes, it appears that when individuals consume a diet that is higher in fat, this can help keep the system running smoothly and will prevent gallstones from forming in the first place.

Improved Kidney Function

Another common issue among the health community is kidney stones. The most common cause of both gout and kidney stones is due to elevated levels of phosphorus, oxalate, calcium, and uric acid in the body. Unfortunately, this is often combined with obesity, dehydration, bad genetics, sugar consumption, and alcohol consumption.

Through the Ketogenic diet, individuals are able to lower their uric acid levels and help improve the health of their kidneys. It should be noted that while the ketogenic diet can help long-term, this diet does temporarily raise the uric acid levels within the body, especially if you are dehydrated. While it does rise as the ketone levels rise, the uric acid levels will lower in about four to six weeks.

Improved Women's Health

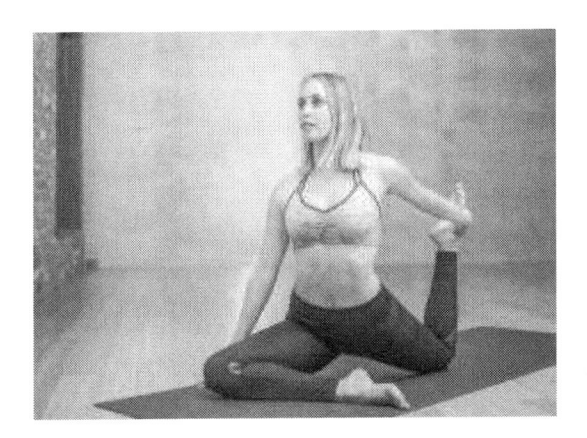

While the ketogenic diet is beneficial for both men and women, studies have shown that through diet, women may be able to stabilize their hormones and increase their fertility.

There was extensive research published in 2013 that looked at the key evidence linking ketogenic diets to enhancing fertility. It was also found that the Ketogenic Diet can treat PCOS (Polycystic Ovary

Syndrome.) Through diet, individuals were able to eliminate or reduce symptoms of PCOS, including obesity, acne, and prolonged menstrual periods.

On a more general basis, it seems as though with this diet, individuals were able to keep their blood sugar levels low and stable. When this happens, it helps stabilize and equilibrate hormone levels, especially in women. Fortunately, this is a downstream benefit of the metabolic pathways that are related to insulin. Overall, individuals feel more balanced and stable than ever!

Improved Endurance and Muscle Gain

As we get older, we generally begin to lose the muscle mass we once had. As mentioned, one of the main ketones you will begin producing as you begin the Ketogenic Diet is BHB. BHB is helpful in promoting muscle gain. When you combine the ketogenic diet with proper exercise, you will be increasing your health and muscle gain at the same time.

In addition to muscle gain, it is also believed that the diet can help improve endurance. Studies have found that athletes who switched to the diet and became fully fat-adapted showed significant improvements in both their mental and physical performances. Of course, this was compared to individuals who followed a typical diet that is rich in carbohydrates.

Weight Loss

Weight loss is one of the major reasons anyone begins a diet. Luckily through the ketogenic diet, there is substantial evidence that by eating the proper foods, you will be able to lose weight and preserve your muscle mass. In a related study, it was found that individuals who followed a ketogenic diet, compared to individuals on a low-calorie and low-fat diet were able to lose 2.2 times more weight! In addition, these people also improved their HDL cholesterol and Triglyceride levels.

The best part about losing weight on the Ketogenic diet is the fact that individuals are still able to lose fat without restricting their calories nor controlling their food intake. This is important to keep in mind when it comes down to sticking to any diet. When individuals hate the extra work of counting their calories, they are statistically more likely to return to their old eating habits.

Increased Metabolic Health

The last health benefit we will focus on increased metabolic health. Metabolic syndrome is described as give common risk factors for heart disease, type 2 diabetes, and obesity. These include high blood sugar levels, low levels of HDL "good" cholesterol, high levels of LDL "bad" cholesterol, abdominal obesity, and high blood pressure. The good news is that many of these risk factors can be eliminated or improved through better lifestyle and nutritional changes. An important factor behind these issues is insulin. Insulin plays a vital role as far as metabolic disease and diabetes go.

Luckily, the Ketogenic Diet is very effective when it comes to lowering insulin levels for individuals who are prediabetic or have type 2 diabetes.

In one study, it was found that after only two weeks following the Ketogenic Diet, individuals were able to improve their insulin sensitivity by 75% and showed a blood sugar level drop from 7.5 mmol/l to a 6.2mmol/l! In another 16-week study, seven out of the 21 participants were able to stop their diabetic medication completely when they began the Ketogenic Diet.

As you can tell, the Ketogenic Diet can help a number of different people. While that is important to know, it is more important to understand how it works. The key to your success is going to be fat! While that may seem backward, what we are taught about fat is all backward! Yes, there are bad fats that we have to avoid, but good fat is going to be your new fuel source.

Chapter 7: Keto Side Effects and How to Solve Them

It would be very irresponsible of me if I only tell you all the good things about the Ketogenic Diet and ignore the side effects. The truth is that there are negative effects that could happen once you start the Ketogenic Diet—but that's actually true for all of them! All types of diet have negative effects to start with because your body has gotten used to the bad habits. Once you make the shift to a more positive way of eating, the body sort of goes on a rebellious phase, so it feels like everything is going wrong. For example, a person who used to eat lots of sugar in a day can have severe headaches once they start to avoid the sugar. This is a withdrawal symptom and tells you that your diet is actually making positive changes to the body—albeit it takes a little bit of pain on your part.

So what can one expect when they make that change towards a healthy Ketogenic Diet? Here are some of the things to expect and of course – how to troubleshoot these problems.

Long Term Side Effects

A study titled "Metabolic Effects of the Very Low Carbohydrate Diets: Misunderstood Villains of Human Metabolism" shows that for short-term purposes, the Ketogenic Diet is very effective. It lets you burn all those excess fat quickly but in a healthy way. If you do this for a long period of time, however, there will be side effects. For example, there can be muscle loss, dizziness, kidney problems, acidosis, and problems with focus. Does that mean you shouldn't go on a Ketogenic Diet at all? Of course not! This only means that you'll have to be careful when using this diet. Don't push it too hard and you will be able to get all the positive results with none of the downsides!

Do you know why a low carbohydrate diet is bad if done for a long time? Well, balance is important in anything you do, and the Ketogenic Diet doesn't really support balance. If you get rid of an entire food group for a long period of time, your body will rebel against you. Remember – the Ketogenic Diet relies on stored fat in your body. If there are no more stored fat, it really won't work anymore so you will have to increase your carbohydrates. To solve this problem, I recommend going on a 30-day Ketogenic Diet first and assessing your health before moving forward. Asking your doctor what to do "next" after the 30-day plan or after hitting your weight goal is also a good idea. Personally, I decided to increase my carbohydrate intake slightly after hitting my goal weight.

Keto Flu

The Keto Flu is the most prominent problem you'll encounter when starting the diet. It's a perfectly normal reaction by the body that may seem alarming because, well, the symptoms don't really feel good. You have to understand, your body has been running on a specific type of gasoline for years. It's been taking fuel from sugar, and with the Ketogenic Diet, it's like you're changing your fuel source to a cleaner and more sustainable type. It makes sense that the engine growls a little in protest—but after that, you'll be able to run beautifully without the guilt.

The Keto Flu has the following symptoms:

- Headaches

- Fatigue

- Irritability

- Brain fog or difficulty focusing

- Motivational problems

- Sugar cravings

- Dizziness

- Nausea

- Muscle cramps

- Frequent urination

These symptoms are all heavily dependent on the kind of person doing the Keto Diet. Since you're already in our 50s, the symptoms may be more prominent, especially if you rely heavily on carbohydrates in your diet. If you eat mostly low-carb food; however, these effects may not be as obvious. But how do you solve them? Here are some of the best way to get rid of the Keto Flu as quickly as possible!

First, increase your water and salt consumption. This happens a lot once you start a Ketogenic Diet. You may not notice it, but a lot of the salt you consume is through carbohydrates like bread, pasta, rice, and so on. Salt tends to make you thirsty, so if you eat little salt, you're also less likely to look for water during the day. So what happens now? Every time you feel dizzy or tired or nauseous while on a Keto Diet, just dissolve salt in water and gulp it down. Now, this is not going to taste good - but I promise that it will help you feel better. You can always try consuming the salt and water separately – whatever you find most convenient. Beef stock, bone broth, or chicken stock are also great alternatives and tastier too! As for water, try to hit a target of 3 liters of water every day. The good news is that this doesn't have to be plain water – your smoothies, coffee, and tea drinks are also counted.

Add more fat in your diet. Because of all the wrong information circulating today, a lot of people are afraid of fat. Fat is not your enemy. During the Ketogenic Diet, it makes sense to eat lots of fats, especially if your carbohydrate intake dips to an all-time low. If you lower the carbohydrate consumption without an equal fat increase, then you will always feel hungry and tired.

Don't be impatient—go slower. Remember what we said about the body changing fuels when you're switching to the Ketogenic Diet? Well, the changing process doesn't have to be overnight. Choose to convert one meal at a time to a Keto-friendly set instead of changing all of them on your first day. Of course, it's recommended that you only do this if the salt water method doesn't work for you. Just remember—The Keto Flu will pass so the first few days of discomfort should not discourage you in the slightest. If you want to minimize the trouble, try starting your Ketogenic Diet on a low-stress period – like a holiday. So basically, instead of eating less than 50 grams of carbohydrates a day, you can have a target of 50 to 70.

Do NOT count calories or restrict your food consumption. When it comes to the Ketogenic Diet—you don't have to calorie count. Again, you don't want to just stuff yourself with food just because you don't have to count calories, but the truth is calories do not matter so much when your body is at a state of Ketosis. It doesn't matter so much how many you're getting—your body will always break down the fat deposits and there will be weight loss. Stressing about the calorie intake or depriving yourself of food because of the calories can actually worsen the symptoms of Keto Flu and will make it more difficult for you to stick to the diet. The bottom line is this: as long as you're eating the allowed food items in allowed portions, then you're OK.

Limit your physical activity. That's the good news with the Ketogenic Diet—you don't have to exercise. Sure, you may not be running marathons or going to the gym on a weekly basis, but if you're health-conscious, then chances are you do light walks on a routine basis. That's perfectly OK—as long as you don't over-exert yourself. Now, there will be days when you will actually feel too good. Like you can go out and exercise because you have all this extra energy. When this happens, resist the temptation to do too much too soon. Your body is already burning as much fat as it can – don't push it too hard or you might get sick. If you're restless, try doing yoga, light walking, or just stretching.

Take some supplements. People using the Ketogenic Diet for a long time may also have vitamin and mineral deficiency. It's not easily obvious, but it could happen so you'll have to be prepared. The usual vitamins and minerals lacking in a Ketogenic Diet include calcium, zinc, selenium, and vitamin D—so try taking a multivitamin during your diet. Again, I can't stress this enough: always consult your doctor before taking any sort of medication. This is especially true if you have pre-existing health problems and are also taking medication for maintenance.

Constipation or Diarrhea

These problems are fairly common because, well, you're changing your diet! Your body will react one way or another, and in both cases, the solution is practically the same—water and fiber. Make sure you get enough fluids in your system and take fiber supplements which is available through many stores. You can also try taking laxatives that are made especially without carbohydrates.

If alarming symptoms occur while you're on the Ketogenic Diet, I want you to consult your doctor ASAP! Again, reactions may vary from one person to the next, and I don't want you shrugging off certain symptoms as if they're just "part" of the diet. Stay motivated but also be mindful of what is happening to your body. Remember—we want you to be healthy!

Chapter 8: Most Common Keto Diet Mistakes You Should Know

The 9 Common Mistakes Beginners Do During Keto

Getting energy from fat, not sugar, is a very good approach and, as we have seen, can bring various health benefits. However, if you keep on the ketogenic diet every day, you can make some mistakes. If you know them, you can avoid them and realize their full potential.

Give up before you stop ketosis

Food ketosis is a mandatory step and has more or less obvious and more or less long-term effects. They vary depending on how much carbohydrate has been abused before and how much our hearts are overloaded. When the body switches from burning sugar to burning fat, we feel like poisoned and weighed. They are poisons that rise and start blooming again after one or two weeks. Other symptoms associated with persistent ketosis include:

- Halitosis
- A little nauseous
- Early hunger for sugar
- Fatigue
- Nervousness
- A little sadness

These last symptoms are related to the effects of sugar and carbohydrate excretion on our mind, which makes us happy and satisfied by stimulating the same opiate receptors.

Conversely, if you stop them now and lose the allure, you might feel a little sad and nervous.

Many are afraid of these symptoms and are not well informed. They believe that the ketogenic diet is not for them, that they are worse off at the start and give up everything before they switch to ketosis.

Lack of salt and minerals

The desire for sugar which was originally accused can be exacerbated by the possibility of mineral deficiencies. Therefore, they need to be integrated with the right dose of potassium, magnesium and sodium. Using Himalayan salt, eating salty snacks, using magnesium in the evening, could be just as many ways to remedy this mistake.

Consume too much protein

At the beginning, higher doses of protein help to overcome hunger crises, but then it is good to go back to consuming the right amount. To know how many proteins we should consume, just multiply our weight by 0.8 if we do normal physical effort and by 1.2 if we are sports. Another mistake regarding this category of food, which generally tends to be made, is that of consuming poor-quality proteins, such as pork, cold cuts or putting different sources of protein on the same plate.

Insufficient fat consumption

This is another mistake that is easy to run into if we follow the ketogenic diet. We continue to be afraid of consuming fats and not using all-natural sources: coconut oil, ghee, MCT oil, egg yolk, fatty fish, butter and avocado. The opposite mistake is to exaggerate with oilseeds: walnuts, almonds, flax seeds, pumpkin seeds that if we neglect to soak in advance with water and lemon, we also absorb the phytic acid they contain, a pro-inflammatory substance and antinutrient.

Consume bad quality food

It is another of the most common mistakes. We focus on weight loss, but continue to consume frozen, canned, highly processed and, as mentioned, proteins that are practical and quick to eat, but of poor quality.

Do not introduce the right amount of fiber

Vegetables should always be fresh and consumed in twice the amount of protein and always cooked intelligently, that is, never subjected to overcooking or too high temperatures. In everyday life, if present, however, we often resort to ready-made, frozen or packaged vegetables. Also with regard to fruit, we often resort to the very sugary one, we forget that there are many berries with a low glycemic index: berries, mulberries, goji berries, Inca berries, maqui.

Eat raw vegetables

I know this may surprise you, but consuming large quantities of raw vegetables, centrifuged, cold smoothies, over time slow down digestion, cool it, undermine our ability to transform food and absorb nutrients. This exposes us over time to inevitable deficiencies: joint pain, teeth, nails and weak hair, anemia, fatigue, abnormal weight loss.

Consume the highest protein load at dinner

This is a mistake that involuntarily, we all commit. The work, the thousand commitments, lead us to stay out all day, to eat a frugal meal for lunch or even not to consume it at all. Here the dinner turns into the only moment of the day in which we find our family members, we have more time, we are more relaxed, and we finally allow ourselves a real meal complete with vegetables, proteins, sometimes even carbohydrates and then fruit or dessert to finish. It escapes us that even the healthiest protein, the freshest or most organic food, weighs down the liver. During the night, this being busy helping digestion, it cannot perform the other precious task: to purify the blood, prepare hormones, energy for the next day.

Not drinking enough

And above all, don't drink hot water. You got it right, drinking hot water is another story entirely, a huge difference from drinking it even at room temperature. The benefits are many: greater digestibility and absorption, deep hydration of cells, brighter skin and hair, retention disappears, cellulite improves, kidneys are strengthened, digestion improves, heartburn subsides.

Ketogenic Foods

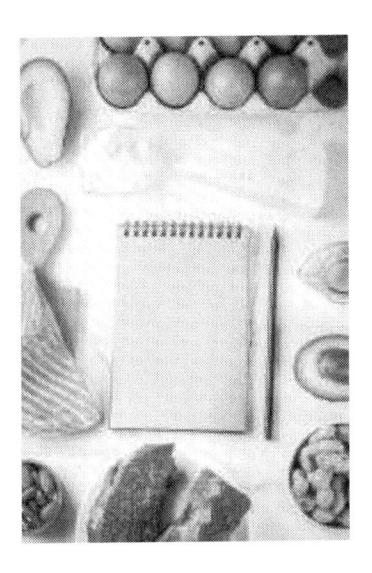

Best Foods to Fit into the Keto Diet for Older Adults

I will go over what food you should consider incorporating into your keto diet. But the general guideline is that all foods that are nutritious and low in carbs are excellent options.

Seafood

Fishes and shellfishes are perfect for keto diets. Many fishes are rich in B vitamins, potassium, as well as selenium. Salmon, sardines, mackerel, and other fatty fish also pack a lot of omega-3 fats that help in regulating insulin levels. These are so low in carbs that it is negligible.

Shellfishes are a different story because some contain very few carbs, whereas others pack plenty. Shrimps and most crabs are okay but beware of other types of shellfish.

Vegetables

Most vegetables pack a lot of nutrients that your body can greatly benefit from even though they are low in calories and carbs. Plus, some of them contain fiber, which helps with your bowel movement. Moreover, your body spends more energy breaking down and digesting food rich in fiber, so it helps with weight loss as well.

Cheese

Milk is not okay. You can get away with cheese though. Cheese is delicious and nutritious. Thankfully, although there are hundreds of types of cheese out there, all of them are low in carbs and full of fat. Eating cheese may even help your muscles and slow down ageing.

Avocados

Avocados are so famous nowadays in the health community that people associate the word "health" to avocados. This is for a very good reason because avocados are very healthy. They pack lots of vitamins and minerals such as potassium. Moreover, avocados are shown to help the body go into ketosis faster.

Meat and Poultry

These two are the staple food in most keto diets. Most of the keto meals revolve around using these two ingredients. This is because they contain no carbs and pack plenty of vitamins and minerals. Moreover, they are a great source of protein.

Eggs

Eggs form the bulk of most food you will eat in a keto diet because they are the healthiest and most versatile food item of them all. Even a large egg contains so little carbs but packs plenty of protein, making it a perfect option for a keto diet.

Moreover, eggs are shown to have an appetite suppression effect, making you feel full for longer as well as regulating blood sugar levels. This leads to lower calorie intake for about a day. Just make sure to eat the entire egg because the nutrients are in the yolk.

Coconut Oil

Coconut oil and other coconut-related products such as coconut milk and coconut powder are perfect for a keto diet. Coconut oil, especially, contain MCTs that are converted into ketones by the liver to be used as an immediate source of energy.

Plain Greek Yogurt and Cottage Cheese

These two food items are rich in protein and a small number of carbs, small enough that you can safely include them into your keto diet. They also help suppress your appetite by making you feel full for longer, and they can be eaten alone and are still delicious.

Olive Oil

Olive oil is very beneficial for your heart because it contains oleic acid that helps decrease heart disease risk factors. Extra-virgin olive oil is also rich in antioxidants. The best thing is that olive oil can be used as a main source of fat and it has no carbs. The same goes for olive.

Nuts and Seeds

These are also low in carbs but rich in fat. They are also healthy and have a lot of nutrients and fiber. They help reduce heart disease, cancer, depression, and other risks of diseases. The fiber in these also help make you feel full for longer, so you would consume fewer calories and your body would spend more calories digesting them.

Berries

Many fruits pack too many carbs that make them unsuitable in a keto diet, but not berries. They are low in carbs and high in fiber. Some of the best berries to include in your diet are blackberries, blueberries, raspberries, and strawberries.

Butter and Cream

These two food items pack plenty of fat and a very small amount of carbs, making them a good option to include in your keto diet.

Shirataki Noodles

If you love noodles and pasta but don't want to give up on them, then shirataki noodles are the perfect alternative. They are rich in water content and pack a lot of fiber, so that means low carbs and calories and hunger suppression.

Unsweetened Coffee and Tea

These two drinks are carb-free, so long as you don't add sugar, milk, or any other sweeteners. Both contain caffeine that improves your metabolism and suppresses your appetite. A word of warning to those who love light coffee and tea lattes, though. They are made with nonfat milk and contain a lot of carbs.

Dark Chocolate and Cocoa Powder

These two food items are delicious and contain antioxidants. Dark chocolate is associated with the reduction of heart disease risk by lowering the blood pressure. Just make sure that you choose only dark chocolate with at least 70% cocoa solids.

Allowed Product List

If you've decided to go on Keto after 50, be sure you won't regret your choice! So when you start something new, the first and the main thing you need to do is consult the Keto dietary features. But most importantly, you must look at the list of allowed products to remember this list and adhere strictly to it.

Don't worry! The low-carb eating plan isn't overly limited. Check out what products you can and must buy in the supermarket and start a new phase in your life.

Meat and Poultry

Chicken, beef, pork, lamb, turkey, veal include no-carb, but high protein and fat intake. That is the primary reason why meat and poultry products are known as the staples for the Ketogenic diet. Besides this, bacon and organ meats are also allowed for consumption.

Seafood

When it comes to seafood, you also have an excellent list. You can buy and cook a lot of delicious dishes from:

- Lobster
- Shrimp
- Octopus
- Salmon
- Tuna
- Oysters
- Mussels
- Squid
- Scallops

The most useful Keto seafood is the crab and shrimp. They don't contain carbohydrates at all.

Vegetables

Only low-carb and non-starchy veggies can be eaten by the people who go on the Keto diet. This means that you can add the following vegetables:

- Avocados
- Tomatoes
- Cucumbers
- Zucchini

- Radishes
- Mushrooms
- Eggplant
- Celery
- Bell peppers
- Herbs
- Asparagus
- Kohlrabi
- Mustard
- Spinach
- Lettuce
- Kale
- Brussel sprouts

Dairy Products

You should be careful with dairy. Not all dairy food can be useful for you if you want to stick to the Keto diet. Here are the products you can buy and cook:

- Eggs

- Butter and ghee

- Heavy cream and whipping cream

- Sour cream

- Unflavored Greek yogurt

- Cottage cheese

- Hard, semi-hard, soft, and cream cheeses

Berries

Unfortunately, most fruits have high levels of carbs and can't be included on the Keto diet. However, you can consume:

- Blackberries

- Raspberries

- Strawberries

- Blueberries

Nuts and Seeds

A lot of experts recommend paying attention to nuts and seeds that are high-fat and low-carb. You can add such nuts and seeds to your dishes as:

- Almond
- Pecans
- Walnuts
- Hazelnuts
- Brazil nuts
- Pumpkin seeds
- Sesame seeds
- Chia seeds
- Flaxseed

Coconut and Olive Oils

To cook tasty fatty dishes, you need oil. Coconut and olive oils have unique properties that make them suitable for a Keto diet. These oils are rich in fat and boost ketone production. Moreover, they can be used for salad dressing and adding to cooked dishes.

Low-Carb Drinks

The Keto diet means that you should drink only unsweetened coffee and tea because they don't include carbs and fasten metabolism. Besides, you can drink dark chocolate and cocoa. Such drinks have low levels of carbohydrates and that's why they're permitted.

Prohibited Product List

When it comes to the lists of foods, you should avoid on the low-carb, high-fat diet, be attentive and check it carefully. Well, you can't eat:

- Grains (like oatmeal, pasta, bulgur, corn, wheat, buckwheat, rice, etc.)
- Low-fat dairy (fat-free yogurt, skim milk, skim Mozzarella, etc.)
- Most fruits (melon, watermelon, apples, peaches, bananas, grapes, oranges, plums, grapefruits, mangos, cherries, pineapples, pears, etc.)
- Starchy veggies (potatoes, beets, turnips, parsnips, etc.)
- Grain foods (pasta, popcorn, muesli, cereal, bagels, bread, etc.)
- Some oils (soyabean oil, grapeseed oil, sunflower oil, peanut oil, canola oil)
- Typical snack foods (crackers, potato chips, etc.)
- Trans fats (margarine)
- Sweets (candies, buns, pastries, cakes, chocolate, puddings, cookies)
- Sweeteners and added sugars (corn syrup, cane sugar, honey, agave nectar, etc.)
- Sweetened drinks (sweetened coffee and tea, juice, soda, smoothies.
- Alcohol (sweet wines, cider, beer, etc.)

Keto diet Menu for The Beginner: Understanding SKD, TKD and CKD

If this spring you've decided to lose weight, then you might want to look at the Keto diet. The diet has been around for a long time and was once used to treat patients with epileptic or seizure disorders, especially in young children. Currently, the diet has lost its prominence with the emergence of prescription drugs to manage the health issue. Nevertheless, the diet is used by many dieters around the world because of its success, and while diets have their side effects, learning about the diet and following the rules will help one lose weight without losing overall health.

In fact, beginners should have a brief overview of their food and meal schedule to aid them in making informed decisions should they decide to take their own diet.

As always, those with health problems should consult their health care provider to help patients adjust to the meal plan or monitor them to ensure that their health is not affected by ketogenic therapy.

Keto diet is a low-carbohydrate high-fat diet with adequate protein in the meal. It is further broken down into three types, and depending on your daily calorie needs, the percentage varies. Diets are often prepared in a 4:1 or 2:1 ratio, with the first number showing the total amount of fat in the diet as compared to the combined protein and carbohydrate in each meal.

Standard-SKD

The first diet is the Standard or SKD and is designed for people who are not active or who lead a lifestyle that is sedentary. The meal plan limits the dieter to eat a carbohydrate net of 20-50 grams. Starchy fruits or vegetables are limited from the diet. To be effective in the diet, the meal plan must be strictly followed. Butter, vegetable oil, and heavy creams are heavily used in the diet to substitute carbohydrates.

Targeted-TKD

The TKD is less stringent than the SKD and allows you to consume carbohydrates but only in a certain portion or quantity that will not affect the ketosis you are currently in. The diet of TKD helps dieters performing some exercise or workout level.

Cyclical-CKD

The CKD is preferable for those undergoing weight training or intensive exercises and not for beginners as it requires the person undergoing the diet to adhere to a five-day SKD meal plan in a week's time and to eat/load carbohydrate over the next two days. It is important for dieters to follow the strict regime to ensure a successful diet.

These are just a brief overview of the keto diet and would hopefully help you decide if you are interested in the diet. It is best to consult your health care provider for an in-depth discussion of the benefits and effects of the diet plan.

Chapter 9: Fitness and Exercise: How to Lose Weight and Alleviate the Symptoms of Menopause

The first aspect that we have seen so far is nutrition. We say that a woman tends to consume less. The first thing we have to do is reduce the kcal that we have introduced. We try to keep a food diary for a week, we record each meal and relative grams, so we include everything in a nutritional application and try to reduce kcal by 5-10% next week.

Let's look at how it works, and if the weight doesn't move, we reduce it by another 5 – 10% so we can reach the desired weight. We come to the second aspect, which is related to training. In this case, women must avoid all activities that can inflame.

Therefore, we avoid many repetitions, but limit ourselves to working with 3 series for each muscle group, 8 to 15 repetitions coming to feel muscle fatigue at the end of each series. This work will enable us to increase muscle tone without inflaming ourselves locally and systemically. Our advice is to exercise at least 2-3 times a week for 45-60 minutes to lose weight during menopause. The first thing you need to know: You need to determine what your goals are. This point is very basic: each physical activity has different characteristics and allows you to achieve different results.

Gymnastic activities with little consideration, often produce results and tasks without stopping. So what are the main goals you need to have in your physical activity plan? I would say at least 3:

- Help you burn more calories, keeping the cardiovascular system in shape

- Help you strengthen the tissues that weaken most, i.e. MUSCLE and BONE

- Help you prevent or solve problems typical of this phase, i.e. muscle pain, arthrosis.

Let's be clear right away: there is NO SINGLE activity that can make you achieve ALL these goals SIMULTANEOUSLY. You need a particular type of activity for each of these goals, and now I will explain just what type of activity. If for reasons of time or otherwise you will not be able to do everything, the world certainly does not fall, but at least you will know the reason why you do not reach a certain goal! In short, if you hoped that "an hour of walking + going to dance on Saturday evening" would have an invigorating effect for the muscles, prepare for a small (or big!) disappointment.

One of the most desired and sought after goals through physical activity is that of slimming.

Losing weight is also one of the most "missed" objectives by the various users. The reason is simple: burning calories with physical activity is hard and time-consuming, consuming too many with nutrition is very easy, painless and even pleasant. To help you with physical activity, you need something that allows you to burn a good number of calories.

Keep in mind that to lose fat, you need to take, on average, about 300 calories less per day than you consume. In an hour of walking at "medium" pace, you consume between 100 and 200 calories. And here is why, for most people, the famous "walks" do not have a significant impact on fat: to have a slimming effect, you should walk at least a couple of hours a day in a row. Walking is relaxing and is good for the cardiovascular system, but if your goal is to lose weight; do your math well!

To get an idea, here is the "average" calorie consumption of various activities, calculated on an hour of activity and for a woman weighing 60 kg: if your weight is greater, keep in mind that consumption increases.

Remember: around 300 calories per day, so around 2000 calories per week. That's why "it's tough", and that's why you can't leave the diet behind.

- Aerobics course: 300 kcal/hour
- Medium speed exercise bike: 400 kcal/hour
- Travel at 8 km / h: 500 kcal/hour
- Swimming: around 500 kcal/hour
- Gardening: around 300 Kcal per hour

Physical activity strengthens muscles and bones

Other changes that women hate? There is clearly muscle loss, especially in the arms and legs. Can this muscle be restored? And how? And what can be done about osteoporosis? So, the answers to these questions are: yes, but it's not easy. And that looks. The reason is simple and to understand it, just focus on these two simple concepts:

- Muscles develop and tone only when asked about strengths

- Bones follow the same principle, that is, the more they strain, the stronger they become to tighten muscles and strengthen bones, you need activities that burden you.

Of course, they must be progressive and controlled overloads, but they are always overloads. Consequently, activities such as swimming, walking or cycling will not help you much: the overload (which is not fatigue, be careful!) To which the muscles are subjected is minimal. In fact, the only activity that allows you to strengthen muscles and strengthen bones is physical activity in the gym.

Physical activity in the gym: recommendations

Physical activity in the gym should overload your muscles: Muscles will "register" and "adapt" to these new needs, will be strengthened. For this to happen, weighing a kilo and twisting with a stick is certainly not enough. Ask the trainer for a special muscle strengthening program.

Physical activity to prevent or treat various problems

Menopausal women who don't have to deal with back or neck pain are counted on the fingers of one hand. Among other things, this problem often complicates physical activity: it is very difficult to lift weights when you suffer from back pain!

Therefore, part of your physical activity plan should aim to increase muscle and joint elasticity.

In this case, targeted stretches are extraordinary activities that you can do with other sports, among them. When you visit the gym, let your trainer show some exercise on important points, or contact a physiotherapist for professional advice. Conclusion: What physical activity should I choose?

If you follow my reasons, you understand one thing: one activity is not enough to reach all goals. And if you understand it correctly, it is not easy to achieve certain goals. It would be ideal to schedule activities throughout the day and throughout the week to cover all different aspects, but most people do not have time. So it's better to focus on what seems to be your main goal:

- Do you want to lose fat? As you have seen, you have to grind kilometers!
- Do you want to tone your muscles? Now you know that you have no alternative to the gym!
- Do you want to solve the ailments first? Devote yourself to stretching and stretching, perhaps with the help of a professional

I understand that you may not like reading certain information: maybe you hate gyms, or you thought that walking half an hour in the evening could have positive effects on fat. Let's find out: Exercise is recommended, but certainly not an obligation! Now you know what physical activity is needed to achieve certain goals.

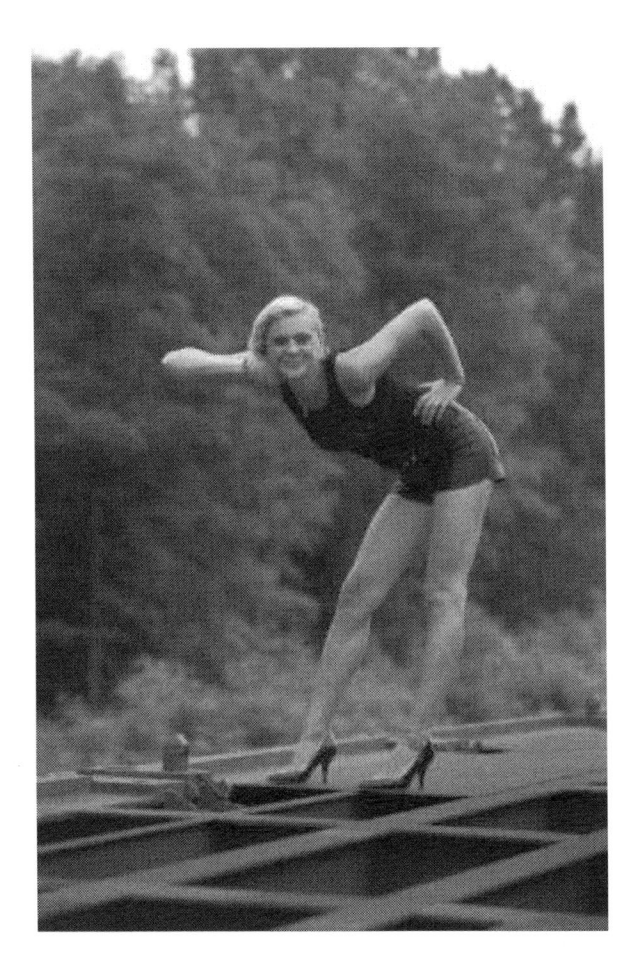

Ketogenic Diet FAQs

Why are you here?

OK —first things first— why are you here? I mean, why are you reading this book? Do you want to lose weight or do you want just to have a healthier lifestyle? This is an important question to ask and in all honesty, I feel like this is a question that we should have addressed in the first stage of the book.

If you'll notice, the book talks about how you can burn fat, lose weight, and prevent diseases with the Ketogenic Diet. Following this dietary plan will give you all three of these results—but finding out your ultimate goal will help you better plan your diet to achieve those goals. For example, if you're already happy with your weight and only want to have a healthier lifestyle, then you don't have to adhere so strictly to the carbohydrate requirement.

This is why I always encourage going to your primary physician first to find out what your dietary limits are. This was the first mistake I made when I decided to follow a weight-loss regiment. Keep in mind—we're trying to improve the quality of your life and not make it worse.

Is there such a thing as too much fat?

Everything in moderation. If you consume too much of one thing, it doesn't matter even if its water—it will be too bad for you. So yes, you can eat too much fat—even if it's healthy fat as already discussed. Remember how we talked about the importance of calories? Well, you have to understand that of all the nutrients found today, fat is perhaps the most compact type. This means that each gram of fat has more calories than any other nutrients you can find today.

What does this mean? This means that if you eat too much fat, there's a good chance that you'll go beyond your calorie requirements. If your goal is weight loss or maintaining a healthy weight, then this is a bad route to take because you won't be experiencing a calorie deficit. Simply put – you'd actually gain weight instead of losing it. I want you to understand this because I don't want you eating more than you should in the mistaken belief that its "healthy" for you.

How much weight can you lose?

The amount of weight you can lose on the Ketogenic Diet depends primarily on how well you stick to the plan. The healthy rate is 2 pounds per week and I strongly recommend that you don't speed it up too much. As mentioned, I lost 30 pounds on the diet—but this took years of hard work and personal research on my part!

Should I be counting calories?

Generally, counting calories is the go-to for people who want to lose weight. You will find, however, that this is not a problem when you're on a Keto Diet. That doesn't mean you should forget calories altogether—it only means that it's not that big of an issue in the grand scheme of things.

So the question is—how many calories should you be eating if you're on a Ketogenic Diet? Well, this depends from one person to the next. You will find that there are calculators that can help you get the proper amount of calories you want to maintain while on Keto. A good online calculator is known as the Mifflin St. Jeor calculator, which allows for a calorie suggestion based on your height, weight, and age.

Of course, if you want to be challenged, here's the typical formula.

For males: 10 multiplied by weight in kilograms + 6.25 x height in centimeters less 5 multiplied by age + 5

For females: 10 multiplied by weight in kilograms + 6.25 x height in centimeters less 5 multiplied by age – 161

Once you get the results, you'll have to multiply it using the following situations:

- Sedentary: x 1.2, if you have minimal physical activities such as having a desk job
- Lightly active: x 1.375 light jogging at least once a week
- Moderately active: x 1.55 moderate activity, at least 6 times a week
- Very active: x 1.725 hard exercise daily or hard exercise twice a week

So it's a little tough—but the online calculator should make the whole thing easier. Generally, however, you'd want to maintain a calorie count of 1500 calories per day for weight loss. For health maintenance without the need to lose weight, you can hit 1800 to 2000 calories – depending on the level of activity you experience every day.

Here's the most important question, however: do you have to be strict about it? The short answer is: YES. Just because you're on the Ketogenic Diet doesn't mean you can eat all the meat you want. This is not a free pass—you still have to be mindful of what you eat.

The good news is that if you follow the Ketogenic Diet strictly, you'll find that the period of satiation is longer. Simply put, you won't feel hungry so quickly on the diet. There will be no mid-afternoon cravings for a snack as you feel full all through the hours between lunch and dinner. Even if you do feel hungry, there are a bunch of Keto-friendly snacks you can reach for.

Primary Keto Guidelines—the Do's and Don'ts of Keto over 50

The Ketogenic Diet isn't as complicated as you would think. The general guidelines are simple and straightforward. Even for someone already in their 50s, the Keto Principle works just as well. Sure, there might be a need to make a few tweaks here and there to guarantee compatibility—but for the most part, everything one needs is easy to access.

What do we mean by that? Well, think about it—a person in their 50s is likely to have several maintenance medicines to help with their health. I know I've been taking several medications to help with problems like blood pressure, blood sugar, and so on. Once I made the decision to start a Ketogenic Diet, all of these medicines have to be taken into consideration. Like, is it OK to limit my food if I'm taking

XXX medicine?

Of course, that's actually just one of the things I had to keep in mind. Here are other things you definitely have to consider when starting this brand new dietary lifestyle.

Do Consult Your Doctor Beforehand

I can't stress this enough—especially for people who fall into a certain age group. Your general practitioner will know your medical history better, your current health status, and whether going on a Ketogenic Diet would be a good idea. It's important to remember that any diet has an impact on things like your mental health and psychological health. The change from a regular carb-full diet to a carb-free one can create pressure on yourself, not just physically and mentally. Simply put, this means that if you're under any sort of stress—the dietary change can do more harm than good. Your general doctor would be able to consider all these factors and give good guidance. At the very least, they can make slight changes to the Ketogenic Diet Principles to meet your health needs.

Do Eat Less Than 50 Grams of Carbohydrates

The whole point of going on a Ketogenic Diet is to force the body to enter that state of Ketosis. To do that, one has to eat less than 50 grams of carbohydrates in a day. To put that in perspective, you should know that a single slice of white bread contains 49 grams of carbohydrates! Hence, people who are used to eating sandwiches for their meals are already eating way beyond the required limit. To let you better understand the low-carbohydrate principle, you should also note that the typical American eats around 225 to 325 grams of carbohydrates every day. For a healthy person with a normal weight, eating carbohydrates of around 225 to 325 is not a problem. For people trying to lose weight; however, this amount should definitely be reduced.

Do Increase Your Fat Intake

When we say fat, we're talking about the healthy kind of fat. Try to stay away from products that are labeled as "fat-free" because this is often packed with starchy ingredients.

Do Eat the Good Kind of Meat

Here's the good news for those following the Ketogenic Diet – meat is your friend. However, meat is your friend only if it's the basic kind. What does this mean? Well, anything processed is not a good idea. You'd want to buy something that's as close to the real thing as possible. Sausages, hotdogs, and other meat products that went through a curing or preservation process are discouraged. If you can buy one directly from the farm, then that would be perfect.

Do Avoid Excessive Exercise

Especially during the first few weeks of keto, try not to exercise or do anything strenuous. I want you to focus on the diet to help yourself better stay faithful to the meal plan. This is because if you push yourself to exercise AND follow the Ketogenic Diet, there's a good chance that you'll fail in both. Pour all your willpower into keeping with the meal plans, even if you only do very little exercise during the week. You will find that even with this approach, you can still lose a significant amount of weight.

The End Goal: Achieving Ketosis

The end goal for the Ketogenic Diet is the same for everyone: achieving that state of Ketosis. That's the time when your body is getting energy from the stored fat instead of the readily-available sugar you eat on a daily basis—but you know about that already.

The real question here is—how do you know you're there? Because weight loss in the Ketogenic Diet may be quick, but it's not that quick! You will be able to observe other changes even before the weight loss begins.

Chapter 10: Keto Recipes

Banana Waffles

Preparation Time: 30 minutes

Cooking Time: 30 minutes

Servings: 4 servings

Ingredient List:

- 4 eggs
- 1 ripe banana
- ¾ cup of coconut milk
- ¾ cup of almond flour
- 1 pinch of salt
- 1 tbsp. of ground psyllium husk powder
- ½ tsp. vanilla extract
- 1 tsp. baking powder
- 1 tsp. of ground cinnamon
- Butter or coconut oil for frying

Directions:

Mash the banana thoroughly until you get a mashed potato consistency.

Add all the other ingredients in and whisk thoroughly to evenly distribute the dry and wet ingredients. You should be able to get a pancake-like consistency

Fry the waffles in a pan or use a waffle maker.

You can serve it with hazelnut spread and fresh berries. Enjoy!

Nutrition: each waffle contains 4g of carbohydrates, 13g fat, 5g protein, and 155 kcalories

Keto Cinnamon Coffee

Preparation Time: 5 minutes

Cooking Time: 5 minutes

Servings: 1 serving

Ingredients:

- 2 tbsp. ground coffee
- 1/3 cup of heavy whipping cream
- 1 tsp. ground cinnamon
- 2 cups water

Directions:

Start by mixing the cinnamon with the ground coffee.

Pour in hot water and do what you usually do when brewing. Use a mixer or whisk to whip the cream 'til you get stiff peaks Serve in a tall mug and put the whipped cream on the surface. Sprinkle with some cinnamon and enjoy.

Nutrition:

1 gram net carb 1 gram fiber   14 grams fat

1 gram protein 136k calories

Keto Waffles and Blueberries

Preparation Time: 15 minutes

Cooking Time: 10 to 15 minutes

Servings: 8

Ingredients:

- 8 eggs
- 5 oz. melted butter
- 1 tsp. vanilla extract
- 2 tsp. baking powder
- 1/3 cup coconut flour
- 3 oz. butter (topping)
- 1 oz. fresh blueberries (topping)

Directions:

Start by mixing the butter and eggs first until you get a smooth batter. Put in the remaining ingredients except those that we'll be using as topping.

Heat your waffle iron to medium temperature and start pouring in the batter for cooking

In a separate bowl, mix the butter and blueberries using a hand mixer. Use this to top off your freshly cooked waffles

Nutrition: 3gnet carbs 5g fiber 56g fat 14g protein 575 kcalories.

Baked Avocado Eggs

Preparation Time: 30 minutes

Cooking Time: 30 minutes max

Servings: 4 servings

Ingredients:

- avocados

- 4 eggs

- ½ cup of bacon bits, around 55 grams

- 2 tbsp. fresh chives, chopped

- 1 sprig of chopped fresh basil, chopped

- 1 cherry tomato, quartered

- Salt and pepper to taste

- Shredded cheddar cheese

Directions:

Start by preheating the oven to 400 degrees Fahrenheit

Slice the avocado and remove the pits. Put them on a baking sheet and crack some eggs onto the center hole of the avocado. If it's too small, just scoop out more of the flesh to make room. Salt and pepper to taste.

Top with bacon bits and bake for 15 minutes. Remove and sprinkle with herbs. Enjoy!

Nutrition: 271calories 21g of fat 7g fat

 5g fiber 13g protein

7g carbohydrates

Mushroom Omelet

Preparation Time: 15 minutes

Cooking Time: 5 minutes

Servings: 1 serving

Ingredients:

- 3 eggs, medium
- 1 oz. shredded cheese
- 1 oz. butter used for frying
- ¼ yellow onion, chopped
- 4 large sliced mushrooms
- Your favorite vegetables, optional
- Salt and pepper to taste

Directions:

Crack and whisk the eggs in a bowl. Add some salt and pepper to taste.

Melt the butter in a pan using low heat. Put in the mushroom and onion, cooking the two until you get that amazing smell.

Pour the egg mix into the pan and allow it to cook on medium heat.

Allow the bottom part to cook before sprinkling the cheese on top of the still-raw portion of the egg.

Carefully pry the edges of the omelet and fold it in half. Allow it to cook for a few more seconds before removing the pan from the heat and sliding it directly onto your plate.

Nutrition:

5 grams of carbohydrates 1 gram of fiber

44 grams of fat

26 grams of protein 520kcalories

Chocolate Sea Salt Smoothie

Preparation Time: 15 minutes

Cooking Time: 5 minutes

Servings: 2 servings

Ingredients:

- 1 avocado (frozen or not)
- 2 cups of almond milk
- 1tbsp tahini
- ¼ cup of cocoa powder
- 1 scoop perfect Keto chocolate base

Directions:

Combine all the ingredients in a high-speed blender and mix until you get a soft smoothie.

Add ice and enjoy! Nutrition:

235 calories 20g fat

11.25 carbohydrates 8g of fiber

5.5g protein

Zucchini Lasagna

Preparation Time: 20 minutes

Cooking Time: 1 hour 20 minutes

Servings: 9 servings Ingredients:

   3 cups raw macadamia nuts or soaked blanched almonds (for ricotta)

2 tbsp. nutritional yeast (for ricotta)

2 tsp dried oregano (for ricotta)

1 tsp. sea salt (for ricotta)

1/2 cup water or more as needed (for ricotta)

1/4 cup vegan parmesan cheese (for ricotta)

1/2 cup fresh basil, chopped (for ricotta)

1 medium lemon, juiced (for ricotta)

Black pepper to taste (for ricotta)

1 28-oz jar favorite marinara sauce

3 medium zucchini squash thinly sliced with a mandolin

Directions:

Preheat the oven to 375 degrees Fahrenheit Put macadamia nuts to a food processor.

Add the remaining ingredients and continue to puree the mixture. You want to create a fine paste.

Taste and adjust the seasonings depending on your personal preferences.

Pour 1 cup of marinara sauce in a baking dish.

Start creating the lasagna layers using thinly sliced zucchini

Scoop small amounts of ricotta mixture on the zucchini and spread it into a thin layer. Continue the layering until you've run out of zucchini or space for it.

Sprinkle parmesan cheese on the topmost layer.

Cover the pan with foil and bake for 45 minutes. Remove the foil and bake for 15 minutes more.

Allow it to cool for 15 minutes before serving. Serve immediately. The lasagna will keep for 3 days in the fridge.

Nutrition:

338 calories 34g fat

10g carbohydrates 5g fiber

4.7g protein

Vegan Keto Scramble

Preparation Time: 15 minutes

Cooking Time: 10 to 15 minutes

Servings: 1 serving

Ingredients:

14 oz. firm tofu

3 tbsp. avocado oil

2 tbsp. yellow onion, diced

1.5 tbsp. nutritional yeast

½ tsp. turmeric

½ tsp. garlic powder

½ tsp. salt

1 cup baby spinach

3 grape tomatoes

3 oz. vegan cheddar cheese

Directions:

Start by squeezing the water out of the tofu block using a clean cloth or a paper towel.

Grab a skillet and put it on medium heat. Sauté the chopped onion in a small amount of avocado oil until it starts to caramelize

Using a potato masher, crumble the tofu on the skillet. Do this thoroughly until the tofu looks a lot like scrambled eggs.

Drizzle some more of the avocado oil onto the mix together with the dry seasonings. Stir thoroughly and evenly distribute the flavor.

Cook under medium heat, occasionally stirring to avoid burning of the tofu. You'd want most of the liquid to evaporate until you get a nice chunk of scrambled tofu. Fold the baby spinach, cheese, and diced tomato. Cook for a few more minutes until the cheese melted. Serve and enjoy!

Nutrition:

212 calories, 17.5g of fat

4.74g of net carbohydrates, 10g of protein

Keto Snacks Recipes

Parmesan Cheese Strips

Preparation Time: 30 minutes

Cooking Time: 30 minutes

Servings: 12 servings

Ingredients:

1 cup shredded parmesan cheese

1 tsp dried basil

Directions:

Preheat the oven to 350 degrees Fahrenheit. Prepare the baking sheet by lining it with parchment paper.

Form small piles of the parmesan cheese on the baking sheet. Flatten it out evenly and then sprinkle dried basil on top of the cheese.

Bake for 5 to 7 minutes or until you get a golden brown color with crispy edges. Take it out, serve, and enjoy!

Nutrition: 31 calories 2g fat

2g protein

Peanut Butter Power Granola

Preparation Time: 30 minutes

Cooking Time: 40 minutes

Servings: 12 servings

Ingredient:

- 1 cup shredded coconut or almond flour
- 1 1/2 cups almonds
- 1 1/2 cups pecans
- 1/3 cup swerve sweetener
- 1/3 cup vanilla whey protein, powder
- 1/3 cup peanut butter
- 1/4 cup sunflower seeds 1/4 cup butter
- 1/4 cup water

Directions:

Preheat the oven to 300 degrees Fahrenheit and prepare a baking sheet with parchment paper

Place the almonds and pecans in a food processor. Put them all in a large bowl and add the sunflower seeds, shredded coconut, vanilla, sweetener, and protein powder.

Melt the peanut butter and butter together in the microwave. Mix the melted butter in the nut mixture and stir it thoroughly until the nuts are well-distributed.

Put in the water to create a lumpy mixture. Scoop out small amounts of the mixture and place it on the baking sheet.

Bake for 30 minutes. Enjoy!

Nutrition: 338kcalories 30g fat 5g carbohydrates9.6g protein 5g fiber

Homemade Graham Crackers

Preparation Time: 15 minutes

Cooking Time: 1 hour 10 minutes

Servings: 10 servings

Ingredients:

- 1 egg, large
- 2 cups almond flour
- 1/3 cup swerve brown
- 2 tsp. cinnamon
- 1 tsp. baking powder
- 2 tbsp. melted butter
- 1 tsp. vanilla extract
- Salt

Directions:

Preheat the oven to 300 degrees Fahrenheit

Grab a bowl and whisk the almond flour, cinnamon, sweetener, baking powder, and salt. Stir all the ingredients together.

Put in the egg, molasses, melted butter, and vanilla extract. Stir until you get a dough-like consistency.

Roll out the dough evenly, making sure that you don't go beyond ¼ of an inch thick. Cut the dough into the shapes you want for cooking. Transfer it on the baking tray

Bake for 20 to 30 minutes until it firms up. Let it cool for 30 minutes outside of the oven and then put them back in for another 30 minutes. Make sure that for the second time putting the biscuit, the temperature is not higher than 200 degrees Fahrenheit. This last step will make the biscuit crispy.

Nutrition:

156kcalories

13.35g fat

6.21g carbohydrates

5.21g protein

2.68g fiber

Keto No-Bake Cookies

Preparation Time: 15 minutes

Cooking Time: 10 minutes

Servings: 18 cook

Ingredient List:

- 2/3 cup of all-natural peanut butter
- 1 cup of all-natural shredded coconut, unsweetened
- 2 tbsp. real butter
- 4 drops of vanilla

Instructions:

Melt the butter in the microwave.

Take it out and put in the peanut butter. Stir thoroughly. Add the sweetener and coconut. Mix.

Spoon it onto a pan lined with parchment paper Freeze for 10 minutes

Cut into preferred slices. Store in an airtight container in the fridge and enjoy whenever.

Nutrition: 80 calories

Swiss Cheese Crunchy Nachos

Preparation Time: 30 minutes

Cooking Time: 20 minutes

Servings: 2 servings

Ingredients:

½ cup shredded Swiss cheese

½ cup shredded cheddar cheese

1/8 cup cooked bacon pieces

Instructions:

Preheat the oven to 300 degrees Fahrenheit and prepare the baking sheet by lining it with parchment paper.

Start by spreading the Swiss cheese on the parchment. Sprinkle it with bacon and then top it off again with the cheese.

Bake until the cheese has melted. This should take around 10 minutes or less.

Allow the cheese to cool before cutting them into triangle strips.

Grab another baking sheet and place the triangle cheese strips on top. Broil them for 2 to 3 minutes so they'll get chunky.

Nutrition: 280 calories per serving

21.8 fat

18.6g protein

2.44g net carbohydrates

Keto Dessert Recipes

Keto Cheesecake with Blueberries

Preparation Time: 30 minutes

Cooking Time: 1 hour 30 minutes

Servings: 12 servings

Ingredients:

1¼ cups almond flour (crust)

2 tbsp. erythritol (crust)

½ tsp of vanilla extract (crust)

2 oz. butter (crust)

20 oz. cream cheese (filling)

2 eggs (filling)

1 egg yolk (filling)

½ cup of crème fraîche or heavy whipping cream (filling)

1 tsp lemon zest (filling)

½ tsp of vanilla extract (filling)

2 oz. fresh blueberries (optional)

Directions:

Preheat the oven to 350 degrees Fahrenheit.

While waiting, prepare a spring form pan by lining it with butter or putting in parchment paper.

Melt the butter until you smell that nutty scent. This will help create a toffee flavor for the crust.

Remove the pan from the heat and add almond flour, vanilla, and the sweetener. Mix the ingredients until you get a dough-like consistency.

Press it into the pan and bake for 8 minutes until you get a slightly golden crust. Set aside to cool.

Now we're going to work on the filling. Mix all the filling ingredients together and beat it heavily. Pour the mixture on the crust.

Increase the oven's heat to 400 degrees Fahrenheit and bake for the next 15 minutes.

Once done, lower it to 230 degrees Fahrenheit and bake again for 45 to 60 minutes

Turn the heat off and leave it inside in the oven to cool.

Remove after it has cooled completely. You can store it in the fridge and serve with fresh blueberries on top.

Nutrition: each slice contains 4g net carbohydrates

33g fat

7g protein

335kcalories

Keto Lemon Ice Cream

Preparation Time: 30 minutes

Cooking Time: 1 hour 30 minutes

Servings: 6 servings Ingredients:

3 eggs

1 lemon, zest and juice

1/3 cup erythritol

1¾ cups heavy whipping cream

Directions:

Grate the lemon to get the zest and then squeeze out the juice. Set it aside in the meantime.

Separate the eggs. Using a hand mixer beat the eggs until they become stiff. Afterwards, beat the egg yolks and sweetener until it becomes light and fluffy.

Add the lemon juice in the egg yolks. Beat it before carefully folding the egg whites into the yolk.

In a separate bowl, whip the cream until you get a soft peak. Gently fold the egg mix into the cream

Pour the whole thing into an ice cream maker and use it according to instructions of the manufacturer.

For those who don't have an ice cream maker, you can just put the bowl in the freezer. You'll have to take it out every 30 minutes to stir it. This should be done for the next two hours until you get the consistency you want.

Nutrition:

27g fat

5g protein

3g net carbohydrates 269kcalories

Peanut Butter Balls

Preparation Time: 30 minutes

Cooking Time: 20 minutes

Servings: 18 servings

Ingredients:

1 cup of salted peanuts chopped finely (not peanut flour)

1 cup of peanut butter

1 cup of sweetener

8 oz. of sugar-free chocolate chips

Directions:

Mix the peanut butter, sweetener, and chopped peanuts together. You'll get a dough-light substance by doing this.

Knead until smooth and then divide the dough into 18 pieces. Shape them into balls.

Place the dough on a baking sheet lined with wax paper before putting them in the fridge to harden.

In the meantime, melt the chocolate chips in a microwave.

Take out the peanut butter balls and dip them in the melted chocolate. Put them back in the fridge to set. Enjoy!

Nutrition:

194kcalories, 17g total fat, 7g carbohydrates, 1g sugar, 7g protein.

Keto Cake Donuts

Preparation Time: 30 minutes

Cooking Time: 30 minutes

Servings: 8 servings

Ingredients:

- 6 eggs
- ½ cup coconut flour
- ¼ tsp. sea salt
- ¼ tsp. baking soda
- 1 tsp. vanilla extract
- ¼ tsp. almond extract
- ½ cup butter or coconut oil
- ½ cup erythritol
- ½ tsp. vanilla extract (frosting)
- ¼ cup melted butter or coconut oil (frosting)
- ¼ cup cream cheese, softened (frosting)
- ¼ cup powdered erythritol (frosting)
- 3 tbsp. melted butter (chocolate drizzle)

2 tbsp. powdered erythritol (chocolate drizzle)

1 tbsp. cocoa powder, unsweetened (chocolate drizzle)

Directions:

Start by preheating the oven to 350 degrees Celsius Fahrenheit Grab a large bowl and out in the donut ingredients.

Take a greased donut pan and will it with batter around 2/3 of the way Bake for 20 minutes.

While waiting, start making the frosting. Do this by putting all the frosting ingredients in a bowl and stir completely with a hand mixer. Add sugar to taste.

Dip the now cool donuts in the frosting and set it on the parchment to cool.

For the chocolate drizzle, put all the ingredients in a small bowl and stir. Drizzle with the liquid as desired.

Nutrition:

294kcalories

2g net carbohydrates 4g fiber

28g fat

6g protein

Chocolate Coconut Candies

Preparation Time: 30 minutes

Cooking Time: 20 minutes

Servings: 20 mini cups

Ingredients:

- 1/2 cup coconut butter
- 1/2 cup Kelapo coconut oil
- 1/2 cup unsweetened shredded coconut
- 3 tbsp. powdered swerve sweetener powdered swerve sweeter
- 1 ½ oz. cocoa butter (topping)
- 1 oz. unsweetened chocolate (topping)
- ½ cup cocoa powder (topping)
- 1/4 cup powdered swerve sweetener (topping)
- 4 tsp vanilla extract (topping)

Directions:

Start by lining the mini muffin with paper liners.

Put the coconut oil and coconut butter in a saucepan and melt it using low heat. Stir completely before adding the shredded coconut and sweetener into the mix.

Divide the mixture onto the mini muffin cups. Set them aside so they'll become firm.

In a separate pan, put cocoa butter and unsweetened chocolate together. Melt them by setting the container in a pan of boiling water. This is done to avoid directly heat on the pan containing the chocolate.

Put the powdered sweetener and cocoa powder slowly until it smoothens into a thick consistency.

Remove it from the heat and put the vanilla extract. Blend carefully.

Spoon the chocolate topping on the firm coconut candies. Wait 15 to 20 minutes for it to set.

Nutrition:

240kcalories

5g carbohydrates 4g of fiber

25g fat

2g protein 6mg sodium

Chicken Wings Black Pepper with Sesame Seeds

Preparation time: 8-10 minutes

Cooking time: 20 minutes

Servings: 2

Ingredients:

- 2 lbs. chicken wings
- 1½ tsps. Salt
- 1½ tsps. black pepper
- 1¼ tbsps. ginger powder
- 1½ tbsps. minced garlic
- 1½ tbsps. extra virgin olive oil
- ½ tbsp. mayonnaise 1 tbsp. sesame seeds

Directions:

Place salt, black pepper, ginger powder, and minced garlic in a bowl then mix well.

Rub the chicken wings with the spice mixture then let them sit for about 5 minutes. Preheat an Air Fryer to 400°F (204°C).

Brush the chicken wings with extra virgin olive oil then arrange in the Air Fryer. Cook the chicken wings for 15 minutes then arrange on a serving dish.

Drizzle mayonnaise over the chicken wings then sprinkles sesame seeds on top.

Serve and enjoy warm.

Nutrition:

Calories: 207 Fat: 16.9g Protein: 7.1g,

Spicy Chicken Curry Samosa

Preparation time: 15 minutes

Cooking time: 30 minutes

Servings: 4

Ingredients:

- 1 lb. ground chicken
- 5 tbsps. extra virgin olive oil
- ¼ c. chopped onion
- ½ tsp. curry powder
- ¼ tsp. turmeric
- ¼ tsp. coriander
- 2 tsps. red chili flakes
- 2 tbsps. diced tomatoes
- ¾ c. almond flour
- ¼ c. water

Directions:

Place ground chicken, chopped onion, curry powder, turmeric, coriander, red chili flakes, and diced tomatoes in a bowl. Mix well. Preheat an Air Fryer to 375°F (191°C) and spray a tbsp. of extra virgin olive in the Air Fryer.

Transfer the ground chicken mixture to the Air Fryer then cook for 10 minutes. Once the chicken is cooked through, transfer from the Air Fryer to a container. Let it cool.

Meanwhile, combine almond flour with 3 tbsps. of olive oil and water then mix until becoming dough. Place the dough on a flat surface then roll until thin. Using a 3-inches circle mold cookies cut the thin dough.

Put 2 tbsps. of chicken on circle dough then fold it. Repeat with the remaining dough and chicken. Preheat an Air Fryer to 400°F (204°C). Brush each chicken samosa with the remaining virgin olive oil then arrange in the Air Fryer.

Cook the chicken samosas for 10 minutes then remove from the Air Fryer. Arrange on a serving dish then serve with homemade tomato sauce or green cayenne.

Enjoy warm.

Nutrition:

Calories: 365 Fat: 30.3g

Protein: 23.1g Carbs: 2.5g

Garlic Chicken Balls

Preparation time: 8-10 minutes

Cooking time: 20 minutes

Servings: 4

Ingredients:

- ½ lb. boneless chicken thighs
- ½ c. chopped mushroom
- 1 tsp. minced garlic
- 1 tsp. pepper
- ½ tsp. salt
- 1¼ c. roasted pecans
- 1 tsp. extra virgin olive oil

Directions:

Cut the boneless chicken into cubes then place in a food processor.

Add roasted pecans to the food processor then season with minced garlic, pepper, and salt. Process until smooth. Cut the mushrooms into very small dices then add to the chicken mixture.

Using your hand mix the chicken with diced mushrooms then shape into small balls. Set aside.

Preheat an Air Fryer to 375°F (191°C).

Brush the balls with extra virgin olive oil then arrange the chicken balls in the Air Fryer. Cook the chicken balls for 18 minutes then arrange on a serving dish.

Serve and enjoy.

Nutrition:
Calories: 525 Fat: 46.8g
Protein: 23.7g Carbs: 5.7g

Savory Chicken Fennel

Preparation time: 15 minutes

Cooking time: 40 minutes

Servings: 4

Ingredients:

- 1½ lbs. chicken thighs
- 2 tsps. fennel
- 1 c. chopped onion
- ¾ tbsp. coconut oil
- 1½ tsp. ginger
- 2½ tsp. minced garlic
- 1½ tsp. smoked paprika
- 1 tsp. curry
- ½ tsp. turmeric
- ½ tsp. salt
- ½ tsp. pepper
- 1½ c. coconut milk

Directions:

Place fennel, chopped onion, and smoked paprika in a bowl.

Season with salt, minced garlic, ginger, curry, pepper, and turmeric then pour coconut oil into the mixture. Mix well. Marinate the chicken thighs with the spice mixture then let them sit for 30 minutes.

After 30 minutes, preheat an Air Fryer to 375°F (191°C).

Transfer the chicken together with the spices to the Air Fryer then cook for 15 minutes. After that, pour coconut milk over the chicken then stir well. Cook the chicken again and set the time to 10 minutes.

Once it is done, arrange the chicken on a serving dish then pour the gravy over the chicken.

Enjoy!

Nutrition:

Calories: 414

Fat: 33.7g

Protein: 22.5g

Carbs: 6.4g

Spicy Glazed Pork Loaf

Preparation time: 15 minutes

Cooking time: 30 minutes

Servings: 8

Ingredients:

- 1½ c. ground pork
- ½ c. diced pork rinds
- ½ tsp. paprika
- ½ tsp. pepper
- 1 tsps. minced garlic
- ½ c. chopped onion
- ½ tsp. cumin
- ½ tsp. cayenne
- ¼ c. butter
- ½ c. tomato puree
- ½ tsp. chili powder
- 2 tbsps. coconut aminos
- ½ tsp. Worcestershire sauce
- 1 tsp. lemon juice

Directions:

Combine ground pork and pork rinds in a bowl then season with paprika, pepper, minced garlic, cumin, cayenne, and chopped onion. Mix well.

Transfer the pork mixture to a silicone loaf pan then spread evenly. Set aside. Next, melt the butter in the microwave then set aside.

Combine the melted butter with tomato puree, chili powder, coconut aminos, Worcestershire sauce, and lemon juice. Stir until incorporated.

Drizzle the glaze mixture over the pork loaf then set aside.

Preheat an Air Fryer to 350°F (177°C). Once the Air Fryer is preheated, place the silicon loaf pan on the Air Fryer's rack then cook for 20 minutes.

Remove from the Air Fryer then let it cool. Cut the pork loaf into slices then serve.

Nutrition:

Calories: 255 Fat: 20.1g

Protein: 13g Carbs: 6g

Spicy Keto Chicken Wings

Preparation time: 20 minutes

Cooking time: 30 minutes

Servings: 4

Ingredients:

- Chicken Wings - 2 Lbs.

- Cajun Spice - 1 t.

- Smoked Paprika - 2 t.

- Turmeric - .50 t.

- Salt - Dash

- Baking Powder - 2 t.

- Pepper - Dash

Directions:

When you first begin the Ketogenic Diet, you may find that you won't be eating the traditional foods that may have made up a majority of your diet in the past. While this is a good thing for your health, you may feel you are missing out! The good news is that there are delicious alternatives that aren't lacking in flavor! To start this recipe, you'll want to prep the stove to 400.

As this heats up, you will want to take some time to dry your chicken wings with a paper towel. This will help remove any excess moisture and get you some nice, crispy wings!

When you are all set, take out a mixing bowl and place all of the seasonings along with the baking powder. If you feel like it, you can adjust the seasoning levels however you would like. Once these are set, go ahead and throw the chicken wings in and coat evenly. If you have one, you'll want to place the wings on a wire rack that is placed over your baking tray. If not, you can just lay them across the baking sheet.

Now that your chicken wings are set, you are going to pop them into the stove for thirty minutes. By the end of this time, the tops of the wings should be crispy. If they are, take them out from the oven and flip them so that you can bake the other side. You will want to cook these for an additional thirty minutes.

Finally, take the tray from the oven and allow to cool slightly before serving up your spiced keto wings. For additional flavor, serve with any of your favorite, keto-friendly dipping sauce.

Nutrition:

Fats: 7g

Carbs: 1g

Proteins: 60g

Cilantro and Lime Creamed Chicken

Preparation time: 10 minutes

Cooking time: 20 minutes

Servings: 4

Ingredients:

- Chicken Breast - 4 Pieces
- Red Pepper Flakes - 1 t.
- Cilantro - 1 T.
- Salt - Dash
- Lime Juice - 2 T.
- Chicken Broth - 1 C.
- Onion - .25 C., Chopped
- Olive Oil - 1 T.
- Heavy Cream - .50 C.
- Pepper - Dash

Directions:

If you are looking for a dish that is a bit different, this recipe is going to be perfect for you. Between the cilantro and the lime, this dish offers a fresh twist on traditional chicken. Many people feel that in order to lose weight, they need to give up flavor, but on the Ketogenic.

Diet, that is simply not the case! To begin this recipe, you will want to get out your cooking skillet and place it over a moderate temperature.

As the skillet heats, go ahead and season the chicken breast according to your taste. For this particular recipe, you will want to consider using the seasonings provided in the list above, but feel free to adjust levels to your own taste. Once seasoned to your liking, throw the chicken into the skillet and cook for about eight minutes on each side. When the chicken is cooked through, take it out of the pan and place to the side.

Next, you are going to add the onion into the hot pan and cook them for a minute before also adding in the cilantro, pepper flakes, lime juice, and the chicken broth. If you don't have chicken broth on hand, feel free to use water. Once these items are in place, bring to a boil for ten minutes.

Last-minute, you are going to whisk in your heavy cream and add in the chicken so that it can be coated in the sauce you just made. For extra flavor, add in some more cilantro, and then your chicken can be served by itself or with a keto-friendly vegetable!

Nutrition:

Fats: 20g

Carbs: 6g

Proteins: 30g

Cheesy Ham Quiche

Preparation time: 10 minutes

Cooking time: 30 minutes

Servings: 6

Ingredients:

- Eggs - 8

- Zucchini - 1 C., Shredded

- Heavy Cream - .50 C.

- Ham - 1 C., Diced

- Mustard - 1 t.

- Salt - Dash

Directions:

Unlike traditional quiche, this version is crustless! Because there is no crust, this recipe offers a low-carb option for those who are still looking to make a savory meal for breakfast or lunch. For this recipe, you can start off by prepping your stove to 375 and getting out a pie plate for your quiche.

Next, it is time to prep the zucchini. First, you will want to go ahead and shred it into small pieces. Once this is complete, take a paper towel and gently squeeze out the excess moisture. This will help avoid a soggy quiche.

When the step from above is complete, you will want to place the zucchini into your pie plate along with the cooked ham pieces and your cheese. Once these items are in place, you will want to whisk the seasonings, cream, and eggs together before pouring it over the top.

Now that your quiche is set, you are going to pop the dish into your stove for about forty minutes. By the end of this time, the egg should be cooked through, and you will be able to insert a knife into the center and have it come out clean.

If the quiche is cooked to your liking, take the dish from the oven and allow it to chill slightly before slicing and serving.

Nutrition:

Fats: 25g

Carbs: 2g

Proteins: 20g

Loaded Cauliflower Rice

Preparation time: 10 minutes

Cooking time: 20 minutes

Servings: 4

Ingredients:

- Cauliflower - 1 Head
- Cheddar Cheese - 1 C.
- Bacon - 1 Lb.
- Chives - .50 C.
- Salt - Dash

Directions:

Sometimes, you just want something basic for lunch. This loaded cauliflower rice is fairly easy to make and only requires a handful of ingredients! The first step of this recipe is going to be ricing your cauliflower. You can choose to do this by hand, or you can purchase cauliflower rice in the frozen section.

Next, you will want to take several moments to cook your bacon. You can complete this task by heating a grilling pan over a moderate temperature and cook the bacon for four or five minutes on either side. I like my bacon crispy, but that is completely up to you!

When you are set, you are going to place your cauliflower rice into a microwave-safe bowl and sprinkle your shredded cheese over the top. When this is set, go ahead and pop the bowl into the microwave for a minute and allow for the rice to cook through and the cheese to melt.

Once the step from above is complete, top the dish off with your bacon pieces and season to your liking. Just like that, lunch will be ready for you!

Nutrition:

Fats: 10g

Carbs: 5g

Proteins: 5g

Super Herbed Fish

Preparation time: 8-10 minutes

Cooking time: 6 minutes

Servings: 1

Ingredients:

- 1 tablespoon chopped basil
- 2 teaspoons lime zest
- 1 tablespoon lime juice
- 1 tablespoon olive oil
- 1 4-ounce fish fillet
- 1 rosemary sprig
- 1 thyme sprig
- 1 teaspoon Dijon mustard
- ¼ teaspoon garlic powder
- Pinch of salt
- Pinch of pepper
- 1 ½ cups water

Directions:

Season the fish with salt and paper. Arrange on a piece of parchment paper and sprinkle with zest.

Whisk together the oil, juice, and mustard in a mixing bowl and brush over. Top with the herbs.

Wrap the fish with the parchment paper. Wrap the wrapped fish in an aluminum foil.

Arrange Instant Pot over a dry platform in your kitchen. Open its top lid and switch it on.

In the pot, pour water. Arrange a trivet or steamer basket inside that came with Instant Pot. Now place/arrange the foil over the trivet/basket. Close the lid to create a locked chamber; make sure that safety valve is in locking position. Find and press "MANUAL" cooking function; timer to 5 minutes with default "HIGH" pressure mode. Allow the pressure to build to cook the ingredients. After cooking time is over press "CANCEL" setting. Find and press "QPR" cooking function. This setting is for quick release of inside pressure. Slowly open the lid, take out the cooked recipe in serving plates or serving bowls, and enjoy the keto recipe.

Nutrition:
Calories: 246
Fat: 9g
Saturated Fat: 1g
Trans Fat: 0g
Carbohydrates: 1g
Fiber: 0.5g
Sodium: 86mg
Protein: 28g

Beef Rib Steak with Parsley Lemon Butter

Preparation time: 8-10 minutes

Cooking time: 40 minutes

Servings: 4

Ingredients:

- 2 beef rib-eye steak
- 2 tbsps. extra virgin olive oil
- ¼ tsp. salt
- ½ tsp. pepper
- ½ c. butter
- ¼ c. chopped fresh parsley
- 2 cloves garlic
- ¼ tsp. grated lemon zest
- 2 tbsps. lemon juice
- 1 tsp. basil
- ¼ tsp. cayenne

Directions:

Brush the beef rib-eye steak with olive oil then sprinkle salt and pepper over the beef. Let it sit for about 30 minutes.

Meanwhile, place butter in a bowl then pours lemon juice over the butter.

Using a fork mix until the butter is smooth. Grate the garlic then add to the butter.

Stir in chopped fresh parsley, grated lemon zest, basil, and cayenne to the butter then mix well. Store in the fridge.

Preheat an Air Fryer to 400°F (204°C) and put a rack in the Air Fryer.

Place the seasoned beef rib eye on the rack then set the time to 15 minutes. Cook the beef.

Once the beef rib eye is ready, remove from the Air Fryer then place on a serving dish.

Serve with the butter sauce. Enjoy right away!

Nutrition:

Calories: 432 Fat: 42.7g

Protein: 10.6g

Carbs: 4.1g

Marinated Flank Steak with Beef Gravy

Preparation time: 8-10 minutes

Cooking time: 20 minutes

Servings: 2

Ingredients:

- 1 flank steak
- ¼ c. butter
- 3½ tbsps. Lemon juice
- 4 tbsps. Minced garlic
- ½ tsp. salt
- ½ tsp. pepper
- c. chopped onion
- ¼ c. beef broth
- 2 tbsps. coconut milk
- 3 tbsps. coconut aminos
- 1 tsp. nutmeg
- 1 scoop Stevia
- 1 tbsp. extra virgin olive oil

Directions:

Allow the butter to melt in the microwave then let it cool.

Combine the melted butter with lemon juice, minced garlic, salt, and pepper then mix well.

Season the flank steak with the spice mixture then marinate for at least 3 hours. Store in the refrigerator to keep it fresh. Preheat a saucepan over medium heat then pour olive oil into the saucepan. Once the oil is hot, stir in chopped onion then sauté until translucent and aromatic. Pour beef broth into the saucepan then season with nutmeg. Bring to boil.

Once it is boiled, reduce the heat then add coconut milk, coconut aminos, and stevia to the saucepan. Stir until dissolved. Get the sauce off heat then let it cool.

After 3 hours, remove the seasoned flank steak from the refrigerator then thaw at room temperature.

Preheat an Air Fryer to 400°F (204°C).
Once the Air Fryer is ready, place the seasoned flank steak in the Air Fryer then set the time to 15 minutes. After 15 minutes, open the Air Fryer then drizzle the beef gravy over the flank steak. Cook the flank steak again and set the time to 5 minutes.

Remove the cooked flank steak from the Air Fryer then place on a serving dish. Drizzle the gravy on top then enjoy right away.

Nutrition:
Calories: 432
Fat: 42.7g
Protein: 10.6g
Carbs: 4.1g

Buttery Beef Loin and Cheese Sauce

Preparation time: 8-10 minutes

Cooking time: 20 minutes

Servings: 3

Ingredients:

- 1 lb. beef loin
- 1 tbsp. butter
- 1 tbsp. minced garlic
- ½ tsp. salt
- ½ tsp. dried parsley
- ¼ tsp. thyme
- ½ c. sour cream
- ¾ c. cream cheese
- 2 tbsps. grated cheddar cheese
- ¼ tsp. pepper
- ¼ tsp. nutmeg

Directions:

Place butter in a microwave-safe bowl then melts the butter. Combine with minced garlic, salt, dried parsley, and thyme then mix well. Cut the beef loin into slices then brush with the butter mixture.

Preheat an Air Fryer to 400°F (204°C). Once the Air Fryer is ready, place the seasoned beef loin in the Air Fryer and set the time to 15 minutes. Cook the beef loin. Meanwhile, place cream cheese in a mixing bowl then using an electric mixer beat until smooth and fluffy. Add sour cream, and grated cheese then seasons with pepper and nutmeg. Beat again until fluffy then store in the fridge.

Once the beef loin is done, remove from the Air Fryer then place on a serving dish. Serve and enjoy with cheese sauce.

Nutrition:

Calories: 441

Fat: 39.4g

Protein: 15.7

Carbs: 5.6g

Chapter 11: Meal Plan

A Keto Diet Meal Plan for women above 5o+ years and Menu that can change your body. The keto diet, generally speaking, is low in carbs, high in fat and moderate in protein. When following a ketogenic diet, carbs are regularly diminished to under 50 grams for every day, however stricter and looser adaptations of the diet exist. Fats supplies most of the carbs and convey roughly 75 percent of your all-out calorie consumption. Proteins should symbolize about 20 percent of vitality, while carbohydrates are generally limited to 5 percent.

The decrease of carbohydrates forces your body to depend on its own energy, which is fats for its primary vitality source to glucose—an event called as ketosis. While in ketosis, your body makes use of ketones—particles delivered to the liver from the fat when glucose is minimized—as another fuel/energy source. Despite the fact that fat is often maintained a strategic distance from for its unhealthy substance, explore shows that ketogenic diets are fundamentally more powerful at advancing weight loss than low-fat diets. In addition, keto diets decrease yearning and increment satiety, which can be especially useful when attempting to get in shape.

Ketogenic Diet Meal Plan

Transferring to a keto diet can show to be overwhelming, yet it doesn't need to be that hard. Your attention should be on minimizing carbohydrates while maximizing the fat and protein substance of meals and bites. In order to be able to maintain ketosis, carbs must be minimized.

While some people may just accomplish ketosis by digesting under 20 grams of carbohydrates every day, some might be fruitful with a lot higher carbohydrates admission. By and large, the lower your sugar admission, the simpler it is to reach and remain in ketosis. This is the reason adhering to keto-accommodating nourishments and maintaining a strategic distance from things rich in carbs is the ideal approach to get thinner on a ketogenic diet effectively.

Weekly Meal Plan (4 Week Meal Plan)

Days	Breakfast	Lunch/Dinner	Snacks
1	Almond, Coconut, Egg Wraps	Cauliflower Mac & Cheese	Chocolate Avocado Ice Cream
2	Bacon & Avocado Omelet	Mushroom & Cauliflower Risotto	Mocha Mousse
3	Bacon & Cheese Frittata	Pita Pizza	Strawberry Rhubarb Custard
4	Bacon & Egg, Breakfast Muffins	Skillet Tacos Cabbage	Creme Brulee
5	Bacon Hash	Taco Casserole	Chocolate

			Avocado Ice Cream
6	Bagels With Cheese	Creamy Salad Chicken	Mocha Mousse
7	Baked Apples	Spicy Keto Chicken Wings	Strawberry Rhubarb Custard
8	Baked Eggs In The Avocado	Cilantro and Lime Creamed Chicken	Creme Brulee
9	Banana Pancakes	Cheesy Quiche Ham	Pumpkin Pudding Pie
10	Breakfast Skillet	Loaded Cauliflower Rice	Vanilla Frozen Yogurt
11	Brunch BLT Wrap	Super Herbed Fish	Ice Cream
12	Cheesy Bacon & Egg Cups	Turkey Chili Avocado	Chocolate Avocado Ice Cream
13	Coconut Porridge Keto	Cheesy Shrimp, Tomato	Mocha Mousse
14	Cream Eggs Cheese	Cajun Chicken, Rosemary	Strawberry Rhubarb Custard
15	Creamy Basil, Baked Sausage	Sriracha Kabobs, Tuna	Creme Brulee
16	Almond, Coconut, Egg Wraps	Chicken Casserole Relleno	Pumpkin Pudding Pie
17	Bacon & Avocado Omelet	Steak Salad with Asian Spice	Chocolate Muffins
18	Bacon & Cheese Frittata	Chicken Chow Mein Stir Fry	Lemon Fat Bombs
19	Bacon & Egg Breakfast Muffins	Choy	Vanilla Frozen Yogurt
20	Bacon Hash	Buttery Garlic Steak	Mocha Mousse

21	Bagels With Cheese	Baked Lemon Salmon	Strawberry Rhubarb Custard
22	Baked Apples	One Sheet Fajitas	Creme Brulee
23	Baked Eggs In The Avocado	Balsamic Chicken	Pumpkin Pudding Pie
24	Banana Pancakes	Cheesy Keto Meatballs	Chocolate Muffins
25	Breakfast Skillet	Beef Rib Steak with Parsley Lemon Butter	Lemon Fat Bombs
26	Brunch BLT Wrap	Marinated Flank Steak with Beef Gravy	Vanilla Frozen Yogurt
27	Cheesy Bacon & Egg Cups	Buttery Beef Loin and Cheese Sauce	Ice Cream
28	Coconut Keto Porridge	Chicken Wings Black Pepper with Sesame Seeds	Chocolate Avocado Ice Cream

Conclusion

Whether you have met your weight loss goals, your life changes, or you simply want to eat whatever you want again, here's the best way to come off the keto diet.

First, you need to prepare yourself mentally. You cannot just suddenly start consuming carbs again, for it will shock your system. Have an idea of what you want to allow back into your consumption slowly. Be familiar with portion sizes and stick to that amount of carbs for the first few times you eat post-keto. Start with non-processed carbs like whole grain, beans, and fruits. Start slow and see how your body responds before resolving to add carbs one meal at a time.

The things to watch out for when coming off keto are weight gain, bloating, more energy, and feeling hungry. The weight gain is nothing to freak out over, perhaps, you might not even gain any. It all depends on your diet, how your body processes carbs, and, of course, water weight. The length of your keto diet is a significant factor in how much weight you have lost, which is caused by the reduction of carbs. The bloating will occur because of the reintroduction of fibrous foods and your body getting used to digesting them again. The bloating van lasts for a few days to a few weeks. You will feel like you have more energy because carbs break down into glucose, which is the body's primary source of fuel. You may also notice better brain function and the ability to work out more.

Printed in Great Britain
by Amazon